A Clinical Guide to Cancer Nursing

JONES AND BARTLETT SERIES IN ONCOLOGY

■ ■ ■

A Clinical Guide to Cancer Nursing

A Companion to *Cancer Nursing, Third Edition*

Edited by

Susan L. Groenwald, RN, MS

Assistant Professor of Nursing—Complemental, Department
of Medical Nursing, Rush University College of Nursing,
Rush-Presbyterian-St. Luke's Medical Center, Chicago, Illinois

Margaret Hansen Frogge, RN, MS

Executive Vice President, Administration; Coordinator,
Community Cancer Program, Riverside Medical Center,
Kankakee, Illinois

Michelle Goodman, RN, MS, OCN

Assistant Professor of Nursing, Rush University College
of Nursing, Oncology Clinical Nurse Specialist,
Section of Medical Oncology, Rush Cancer Institute,
Rush-Presbyterian-St. Luke's Medical Center, Chicago, Illinois

Connie Henke Yarbro, RN, BSN

Editor, *Seminars in Oncology Nursing*
Director, Nursing Resource Development,
The Regional Cancer Center, Memorial Medical Center,
Springfield, Illinois

JONES AND BARTLETT PUBLISHERS
Boston   **London**

Editorial, Sales, and Customer Service Offices
Jones and Bartlett Publishers
One Exeter Plaza
Boston, MA 02116
1-800-832-0034
617-859-3900

Jones and Bartlett Publishers International
7 Melrose Terrace
London W6 7RL
England

Library of Congress Cataloging-in-Publication Data

A clinical guide to cancer nursing : a companion to Cancer nursing,
    third edition / edited by Susan L. Groenwald . . . [et al.].
        p.   cm. —(Jones and Bartlett series in oncology)
    Companion v. to: Cancer nursing / edited by Susan L.
Groenwald . . . [et al.]. 3rd ed. c1993.
    Includes bibliographical references and index.
    ISBN 0–86720–708–6
    1. Cancer—Nursing—Handbooks. manuals. etc.
I. Groenwald, Susan L.   II. Cancer nursing.   III. Series.
    [DNLM: 1. Neoplasms—nursing.   2. Oncologic Nursing—
methods.   WY 156 C6413 1995]
RC266.C55   1995
610.73´698—dc20
DNLM/DLC
for Library of Congress   95–180
                                                                         CIP

The selection and dosage of drugs presented in this book are in
accord with standards accepted at the time of publication. The edi-
tors and the publisher have made every effort to provide accurate
information. However, research, clinical practice, and government
regulations often change the accepted standard in this field. Before
administering any drug, the reader is advised to check the manufac-
turer's product information sheet for the most up-to-date recommendations on dosage, precautions, and contraindications. This is
especially important in the case of drugs that are new or seldom used.

Printed in the United States of America
99   98   97   96   95   10 9 8 7 6 5 4 3 2

Contents

■ PART I ■
The Cancer Problem

■ PART II ■
Diagnosis and Treatment

■ PART III ■
Psychological and Social Dimensions of Cancer

■ PART IV ■
Manifestations of Cancer and Its Treatment

■ PART V ■
The Care of Individuals with Cancer

■ PART VI ■
Delivery Systems for Cancer Care

■ PART VII ■
Professional Issues for the Cancer Nurse

Preface

In our continuing commitment to provide resources to all nurses who come in contact with individuals with cancer, we designed *A Clinical Guide to Cancer Nursing* as an easy-to-use general nursing reference. Information most pertinent to the care of individuals with cancer has been gleaned from *Cancer Nursing: Principles and Practice, Third Edition*, and consolidated in a pocket-size clinical reference.

The content of this clinical guide follows the general outline of *Cancer Nursing: Principles and Practice, Third Edition*. Some chapters were deleted, and other chapters were split into smaller, more specific topics. In Part IV, Manifestations of Cancer and Its Treatment, and Part V, The Care of Individuals with Cancer, chapters were alphabetized by subject for easier access by the reader.

Color and variety of type styles have been used to enhance the readability and aid in locating desired information. Suggested readings have been included to direct the reader to more comprehensive information on the subject, including reference to the chapters in *Cancer Nursing: Principles and Practice* from which the content was extrapolated.

We sincerely hope that this book will be an easy-to-use, quick, and helpful reference to nurses—wherever they are caring for people with cancer.

Acknowledgments

Our special thanks to the nurses who continue to provide us with feedback, suggestions, and encouragement regarding the information and resources they need in caring for patients with cancer. Thanks to Clayton Jones, Jan Wall, and Paul Prindle of Jones and Bartlett for their assistance and their commitment to providing quality textbooks to oncology nurses. Finally, we acknowledge and thank the following authors whose chapters in *Cancer Nursing: Principles and Practice, Third Edition* were used to derive the content contained in this guide:

Connie Yuska Bildstein,
   RN, MS
Northwestern Memorial
   Hospital
Chicago, IL
Head and Neck Cancers

Deborah McCaffrey Boyle,
   RN, MSN, OCN
Fairfax Hospital
Falls Church, VA
Survivorship

Donald P. Braun, PhD
Rush-Presbyterian-St.
   Luke's Medical Center
Chicago, IL
*The Immune System and
   Cancer*

Patricia C. Buchsel, RN,
   MSN
University of Washington
Seattle, WA
*Bone Marrow
   Transplantation*

Dawn Camp-Sorrell, RN,
   MSN, FNP, OCN
University of Alabama
   Hospitals and Clinics
Birmingham, AL
*Toxicity Management in
   Chemotherapy*

Brenda Cartmel, PhD
Arizona Cancer Center,
   University of Arizona
Tucson, AZ
Epidemiology

Dianne D. Chapman, RN, MS
Rush Cancer Institute
Chicago, IL
Breast Cancer

Jane C. Clark, RN, MN, OCN
Emory University Hospital
Atlanta, GA
Psychosocial Dimensions

Kathleen A. Dietz, RN, MA, MS
Memorial Sloan-Kettering Cancer Center
New York, NY
Oncologic Emergencies

Michele Girard Donehower, RN, MSN
University of Maryland Cancer Center
Baltimore, MD
Endocrine Cancers

Henry J. Duravage, PharmD
Theradex
Princeton, NJ
Principles of Chemotherapy

Jan M. Ellerhorst-Ryan, RN, MSN, CS
Critical Care America
Cincinnati, OH
Infection

Ellen Heid Elpern, RN, MSN
Illinois Masonic Hospital
Chicago, IL
Lung Cancer

Betty R. Ferrell, RN, PhD, FAAN
City of Hope National Medical Center
Duarte, CA
Continuity of Care

Anne Marie Flaherty, RN, MS
Memorial Sloan-Kettering Cancer Center
New York, NY
Oncologic Emergencies

Margaret Hansen Frogge, RN, MS
Riverside Medical Center
Kankakee, IL
Esophageal Cancers
Stomach Cancers
Liver Cancer
Pancreatic Cancer

Sue L. Frymark, RN, BS
Good Samaritan Hospital and Medical Center
Portland, OR
Rehabilitation

Barbara Holmes Gobel, RN,
    MS
Lake Forest Hospital
Chicago, IL
Bleeding Disorders

Michelle Goodman, RN,
    MS, OCN
Rush Cancer Institute
Chicago, IL
Breast Cancer
Integumentary Alterations
Mucous Membrane Alterations

Betty Greig, RN, CETN
Kenneth Norris Jr. Cancer
    Hospital and Research
    Institute
Los Angeles, CA
Urologic and Male Genital
    Malignancies

Susan L. Groenwald, RN, MS
Rush-Presbyterian-St.
    Luke's Medical Center
Chicago, IL
Differences Between Normal
    and Cancer Cells
Invasion and Metastasis
The Immune System and
    Cancer
Nutritional Disturbances

Robin R. Gwin, RN, MN,
    OCN
Emory University Clinic
Atlanta, GA
Psychosocial Dimensions

Beverly Hampton, RN, MS,
    ET
M.D. Anderson Cancer
    Hospital
Houston, TX
Colorectal Cancer

Laura J. Hilderley, RN, MS
Private Practice of Philip G.
    Maddock, MD
Warwick, RI
Radiation Therapy

Barbara Hoffman, JD
Private Consultant: Cancer
    Survivorship and
    Discrimination
Princeton, NJ
Survivorship

Patricia F. Jassak, RN, MS,
    CS, OCN
Loyola University Medical
    Center
Maywood, IL
Biotherapy

Barbara Kalinowski, RN,
    MSN, OCN
Faulkner Breast Centre
Boston, MA
Surgical Therapy

Marsha Ketchum, RN, OCN
Arizona Cancer Center,
    University of Arizona
Tucson, AZ
Skin Cancers

Paula R. Klemm, RN,
DNSc, OCN
University of Delaware
College of Nursing
Newark, DE
Gynecologic Cancers

M. Tish Knobf, RN, MSN,
FAAN
Yale-New Haven Hospital
New Haven, CT
Principles of Chemotherapy

Kathy Kravitz, RN, MS
North Colorado Medical
Center
Greeley, CO
*Urologic and Male Genital
Cancers*

Lori A. Ladd, RN, MSN
H. Lee Moffett Cancer Center
and Research Institute
Tampa, FL
*Integumentary Alterations
Mucous Membrane Alterations*

Jennifer M. Lang-Kummer,
RN, MN
East Carolina University
Greenville, NC
Hypercalcemia

Susan Leigh, RN, BSN
Cancer Survivorship
Consultant
Tucson, AZ
Survivorship

Julena Lind, RN, PhD
University of Southern
California
Los Angeles, CA
*Urologic and Male Genital
Cancers*

Lois J. Loescher, RN, MS
Arizona Cancer Center,
University of Arizona
Tucson, AZ
*Survivorship
Skin Cancers*

Jeanne Martinez, RN, MPH
Northwestern Memorial
Hospice Program
Chicago, IL
Hospice

Mary B. Maxwell, RN, CS, PhD
Veterans' Administration
Medical Center
Portland, OR
*Principles of Therapy
Malignant Effusions*

Deborah K. Mayer, RN,
MSN, OCN
Ontario Cancer Institute
Toronto, Ontario, Canada
Rehabilitation

Mary Ellen McFadden, RN,
MLA, OCN
Baltimore, MD
*Malignant Lymphoma
Hodgkin's Disease*

Rose F. McGee, RN, PhD
Nell Hodgson Woodruff
  School of Nursing
Emory University
Atlanta, GA
Psychosocial Dimensions

Deborah B. McGuire, RN,
  PhD, FAAN
Nell Hodgson Woodruff
  School of Nursing
Emory University
Atlanta, GA
Pain

Joan C. McNally, RN, MSN,
  OCN
Michigan Cancer
  Foundation
Detroit, MI
Home Care

Theresa A. Moran, RN, MS
University of California
San Francisco, CA
AIDS-Related Malignancies

Lillian M. Nail, RN, PhD
University of Utah College
  of Nursing
Salt Lake City, UT
Fatigue

Sharon Saldin O'Mary, RN,
  MN
Scripps Memorial Hospital
La Jolla, CA
Diagnostic Measures

Edith O'Neil-Page, RN, BS
Hoag Memorial Hospital
  Presbyterian
Newport Beach, CA
Continuity of Care

Diane M. Otte, RN, MS, ET
St. Luke's Hospital Cancer
  Center
Davenport, IA
Ambulatory Care

Patricia A. Piasecki, RN, MS
Rush-Presbyterian-St.
  Luke's Medical Center
Chicago, IL
Bone Cancers

Sandra Purl, RN, MS, OCN
Rush Cancer Institute
Chicago, IL
Integumentary Alterations
Mucous Membrane
  Alterations

Mary Reid, RN, MPH
University of Arizona
Tuscon, AZ
Epidemiology

Patricia E. Reymann, RN,
  MSN, OCN
Princeton Baptist Medical
  Center
Birmingham, AL
Principles of Chemotherapy
  Administration

Vivian R. Sheidler, RN, MS
The Johns Hopkins
  Oncology Center
Baltimore, MD
Pain

Carol A. Sheridan, RN,
  MSN, OCN
Montefiore Medical Center
Bronx, NY
Multiple Myeloma

Annalynn Skipper, RD, MS,
  CNSD
Rush-Presbyterian-St.
  Luke's Medical Center
Chicago, IL
Nutritional Disturbances

Debra J. Szeluga, RD, MD,
  PhD
The Johns Hopkins Medical
  Center
Baltimore, MD
Nutritional Disturbances

David C. Thomasma, PhD
Loyola University of
  Chicago Medical Center
Maywood, IL
Ethical Issues

Steven Wagner, RN, BSN
Northwestern Memorial
  Hospice Program
Chicago, IL
Hospice

Janet Ruth Walczak, RN, MSN
The Johns Hopkins
  Oncology Center
Baltimore, MD
Gynecologic Cancers

Jo Ann Wegmann, RN, PhD
California State University
Carson, CA
CNS Malignancies

Maryl L. Winningham, RN,
  PhD, FACSM
University of Utah College
  of Nursing
Salt Lake City, UT
Fatigue

Debra Wujcik, RN, MSN,
  OCN
Vanderbilt Cancer Center
Vanderbilt University
Nashville, TN
Leukemia

Connie Henke Yarbro, RN,
  BSN
Regional Cancer Center
Memorial Medical Center
Springfield, IL
*Questionable Methods of
  Cancer Treatment*

John W. Yarbro, MD, PhD
Regional Cancer Center
Memorial Medical Center
Springfield, IL
Carcinogenesis

PART I

The Cancer Problem

■ 1 ■
Cancer Epidemiology

Overview

- ■ Cancer epidemiology is the study of
1. Frequency of cancer in populations
2. Risk factors
3. Interrelationships between host and environment

Cancer Causation Factors

- ■ **Environment**

1. **Tobacco**
    - ❑ *Most important known cause of cancer*
    - ❑ *Causes about 30% of cancer deaths*
    - ❑ *Cigarette smoking causes 90% of lung cancers*

2. Diet

❏ *Contributing factor in 20% to 70% of cancer deaths*

❏ *A modifiable risk factor*

3. Alcohol

❏ *Associated with cancers of the oral cavity, pharynx, larynx, esophagus, and liver*

❏ *Attributable to 3% of cancer deaths*

❏ *May be synergistic with smoking*

4. Occupational exposure to carcinogens

❏ *Accounts for 4% to 9% of cancer deaths*
❏ *Related primarily to lung cancer*

5. Pollution

❏ *Accounts for 1% to 5% of cancer deaths*
❏ *Related primarily to lung and skin cancers*

6. Reproductive factors and sexual behavior

❏ *Endometrial, breast, and ovarian cancers related to unopposed estrogens*

❏ *Cervical cancer related to number of sexual partners*

7. Viruses

❏ *Account for 15% of worldwide cancer incidence*

❏ *Implicated viruses include*
  □ Hepatitis B virus
  □ Human T-lymphotropic virus type 1
  □ Epstein-Barr virus
  □ Human papillomavirus

8. Radiation

❑ *Responsible for 3% of cancer deaths*

❑ *Types of radiation*
  ☐ Ionizing   ☐ Nonionizing
  ☐ Ultraviolet

9. Antineoplastic drugs

❑ *Second malignancy is late effect of resulting cell damage*

▪ Host factors

1. Age

❑ *Individuals over age 65 are 10 times more likely to develop cancer because of*
  ☐ Prolonged lifetime exposure to cancer-inducing agents
  ☐ Declining efficacy of immune system

2. Genetic predisposition

❑ *Associated with certain types of cancer, such as familial polyposis*

❑ *Aggregates in families due to inherited susceptibility or to common environmental exposure*

3. Ethnicity and race

❑ *Biologic and cultural factors cause differences in incidence and mortality*

4. Socioeconomic status (SES)

❑ *Low SES associated with some cancers, independent of race*

❑ *Strongly associated with lifestyle*

Application to Cancer Nursing Practice

■ **Epidemiologic data are used by nurses to**

1. **Identify high-risk patient populations**

2. **Develop and evaluate effectiveness of cancer prevention programs**

3. **Understand survival rates**
   - ❏ *Calculation of the probability that an individual with a specific disease will be alive at a particular time after diagnosis (usually five years)*

Suggested Readings

1. Cartmel B, Loescher LJ, Villar-Werstler P: Professional and consumer concerns about the environment, lifestyle and cancer. *Semin Oncol Nurs* 8(1):20–29, 1992.

2. Cartmel B, Reid M: Cancer control and epidemiology. In Groenwald SL, Frogge MH, Goodman M, Yarbro CH (eds.): *Cancer Nursing: Principles and Practice* (3rd ed.). Boston: Jones and Bartlett, 1993, pp. 3–27.

3. Oleske DM: Epidemiologic principles for nursing practice: Assessing the cancer problem and planning its control. In Baird SB, McCorkle R, Grant M (eds.): *Cancer Nursing: A Comprehensive Textbook.* Philadelphia: Saunders, 1991, pp. 91–103.

2

Carcinogenesis

Multistage Carcinogenesis

■ Initiation

1. Irreversible first stage of carcinogenesis

2. Carcinogenic agent damages cell's DNA

■ Promotion

1. Reversible second stage of carcinogenesis

2. Involves stimulation of cellular proliferation, rather than damage to DNA

3. Exhibits distinct dose response and measurable threshold

■ Progression

1. Third stage of carcinogenesis

2. Leads to morphologic change and increased grades of malignant behavior

Genes

■ **Oncogenes**

1. Code for cellular growth

2. Alterations by carcinogens such as viruses, chemicals, and radiation "turn on" cell division leading to neoplastic growth

■ **Anti-oncogenes**

1. Called *cancer suppressor genes*

2. Have the opposite function of oncogenes

3. "Turn off" cell division

4. Inhibit malignant growth

■ **Cancers result from combination of absence of cancer suppressor genes and presence of abnormal products of oncogenes**

Examples of Human Tumor Carcinogenesis

■ **Familial cancer**

1. **In some diseases, defective genes are inherited**
   - ❏ *Hereditary retinoblastoma*
   - ❏ *Breast cancer*
   - ❏ *Familial polyposis coli*
   - ❏ *Cancer family syndrome*
   - ❏ *Multiple endocrine neoplasia syndromes*

■ **Viral carcinogens**

1. **Only clearly established human tumor attributable to a virus is T-cell leukemia-lymphoma from human T-lymphotropic virus type 1**

2. **Other tumors associated with viruses include**
   - ❑ *Hairy-cell leukemia*
   - ❑ *Retinoblastoma*
   - ❑ *Cervical carcinoma*
   - ❑ *Hepatocellular carcinoma*
   - ❑ *Burkitt's lymphoma*

■ **Physical carcinogens**

1. **Exert destructive actions on DNA of genes by physical means rather than chemical means**
   - ❑ *Radiation*
   - ❑ *Asbestos*

■ **Chemical carcinogens**

1. **There are few chemicals for which there is strong evidence of cancer causation in humans**
   - ❑ *Tobacco*
   - ❑ *Vinyl chloride*
   - ❑ *Metals*
   - ❑ *Benzene*
   - ❑ *2-Naphthylamine*

3. **Only 4% of cancer deaths in America from occupational exposure**

4. **Chemotherapeutic agents are associated with subsequent development of cancer, especially leukemia and myeloproliferative syndromes**

Suggested Readings

1. Ames BN: What are the major carcinogens in the etiology of human cancer? Environmental pollution, natural carcinogens, and the causes of human cancer: Six errors. In DeVita VT, Hellman S, Rosenberg SA (eds.): *Important Advances in Oncology 1989*. Philadelphia: Lippincott, 1989, pp. 237–247.

2. Brugge J, Curran T, Harlow E, et al (eds.): *Origins of Human Cancer*. Cold Spring Harbor, NY: Laboratory Press, 1991.

3. McMillan SC: Carcinogenesis. *Semin Oncol Nurs* 8(1):10–19, 1992.

4. Yarbro JW: Milestones in our understanding of the causes of cancer. In Groenwald SL, Frogge MH, Goodman M, Yarbro C, (eds.): *Cancer Nursing: Principles and Practice* (3rd ed.). Boston: Jones and Bartlett, 1993, pp. 28–46.

∎ 3 ∎
Differences Between Normal Cells and Cancer Cells

Differences in Growth

- **Primary feature of cancer cell is uncontrolled growth**

1. Normal cells are carefully regulated; number of new cells formed in tissues equals number lost by cell death or injury

2. In cancer, cells continue to divide without regard to needs of host

- **Average human neoplasm doubles in size every 2 months**

1. Cell cycle time of cancer cells is not much different from that of normal cells

2. Number of new cells is greater than number of cells lost, resulting in tumor mass

■ Uncontrolled growth of tumors occurs from

1. Cancer cell immortality

❏ *Most normal cells divide only approximately 50 to 60 times before they die; cancer cells are immortal*

2. Loss of contact inhibition

❏ *When placed in a petri dish, normal cells in culture divide until they form a single layer of cells on the bottom of the culture dish, where they stop dividing*

❏ *Cancer cells do not stop dividing; they pile on top of each other in an unorganized mass*

3. Diminished growth factor requirements

❏ *Cancer cells appear to*

  □ Divide without or with lower concentrations of normal serum growth factors

  □ Make their own growth factors

4. Ability to divide without anchorage to a surface

❏ *Most normal cells will not divide in liquid medium or in suspension surface; they require anchorage to surface to divide*

❏ *Cancer cells grow in suspension or gel*

5. Loss of restriction point in cell cycle

❏ *"Decision" of cell to enter G_0 (resting phase) of cell cycle, or to continue into G_1 occurs at point in G_1 called the* restriction point

❏ *G_0 provides controls over cell division*

❑ *When cell passes restriction point, it is committed to cell division*

❑ *Cancer cells do not have this control, and therefore do not enter G_0*

Differences in Appearance

■ **Normal cells have well-organized and extensive cytoskeleton providing cell structure and shape**

■ **Transformed cells have**

1. **Variable sizes and shapes**
2. **Darker-staining nuclei (hyperchromatism)**
3. **Larger nuclei**
4. **Variety of abnormal mitotic figures**

Differences in Differentiation

■ *Differentiation:* **Process by which cells become specialized for specific functions**

1. **All cells derive from one cell**
2. **Occurs by "turning on and off" of certain genes**
3. **The more differentiated a cell, the more its potential is restricted**
4. **Fully differentiated cells are often incapable of replicating**

■ Cancer cells may arise at any point in differentiation

■ Oncogenes active in embryos but suppressed during differentiation can be reactivated by carcinogenic agents

■ Cancer cells tend to be less differentiated than cells from normal tissue

■ Anaplasia occurs when cancer cells are so undifferentiated that tissue of origin cannot be identified

■ During shift from normal to undifferentiated cells, a sequence of tissue alterations occurs

1. Metaplasia

2. Dysplasia

3. Carcinoma in situ

4. Invasive carcinoma

Differences in Cell Surface

■ Cell membranes of animal cells determine which molecules can enter and leave cell

■ Numerous changes take place in cancer cell surface

1. Glycoproteins are missing or altered

2. Absence of fibronectin prevents cancer cells from attaching to other surfaces

3. Secretion of proteolytic enzymes promotes metastasis

4. **Content and complexity of cell surface glycolipids are reduced**
   - ❑ *Increases responsiveness of cancer cells to growth factors*
   - ❑ *Reduces cell-cell recognition by altering glycolipid surface markers*

5. **Tumor-associated antigens appear on surface of cancer cells**
   - ❑ *Used as tumor markers in*
     - ☐ Cancer detection
     - ☐ Monitoring prognosis
     - ☐ Evaluating treatment measures

6. **Permeability and rate of transport of materials across cell membrane are increased**

Biochemical Differences

■ **Biochemical substances are altered, missing, abnormally secreted, or secreted in increased amounts by tumor cells**

1. **Altered biochemical substances include**
   - ❑ *Cyclic adenosine monophosphate*
   - ❑ *Cyclic guanosine monophosphate*
   - ❑ *Nutrients*
   - ❑ *Chalones*
   - ❑ *Growth factors*

2. **Cell growth and cell-cell interactions are affected**

Genetic Differences

- Cancer arises from single altered cell that acquires heritable and selective growth advantage over other cells

1. Each daughter cell inherits genetic defect
2. Tumor cells are genetically unstable
3. Tumor progression results from additional mutations in cells within clone
4. Result is sequential appearance within tumor of subpopulations of heterogeneous cells

- Tumor heterogeneity identified as most significant cause of cancer treatment failure

Suggested Readings

1. Clark WH: Tumor progression and the nature of cancer. *Br J Cancer* 64:631–644, 1991.

2. Groenwald SL: Differences between normal and cancer cells. In Groenwald SL, Frogge MH, Goodman M, Yarbro C, (eds.): *Cancer Nursing: Principles and Practice* (3rd ed.). Boston: Jones and Bartlett, 1993, pp. 47–57.

3. Groenwald SL: The behavior of malignancies. In Gross J, Johnson BJ (eds.): *Handbook of Oncology Nursing* (2nd ed.). Boston: Jones and Bartlett, 1994, pp. 3–20.

4. Lind J: Tumor cell growth and cell kinetics. *Semin Oncol Nurs* 8(1):3–9, 1992.

■ 4 ■
Invasion and Metastasis

Overview

- Metastasis is most frequent cause of cancer treatment failure
- Up to 60% of individuals with solid tumors have undetected metastasis at diagnosis

Factors Contributing to Metastatic Potential

- Tumor factors

1. Oncogene expression is correlated with metastatic behavior

2. Heterogeneity
   - ❏ *Clones of cells isolated from tumors vary in metastatic potential*
   - ❏ *Metastatic subpopulation dominates tumor mass early in its development*

❑ *Even if 99.9% cell kill is achieved with therapy, for a 1-cm lesion, a significant number (10^6) will remain and continue growing*

❑ *Heterogeneity explains differences in growth and metastasis of similar tumors in different individuals*

3. Production of growth factors

❑ *May signal subpopulations of metastatic cells to proliferate and diversify*

4. Production of angiogenic factors

❑ *Assists metastatic clones to establish blood supply*

5. Motility factors

❑ *Necessary for tumor cells to move away from primary tumor site*

6. Specific cell-surface receptors

❑ *Integrins are crucial for binding of fibronectin and laminin to basement membrane*

7. Invasiveness

❑ *Normal, healthy basement membranes are intact, continuous, and impervious to particles*

❑ *Tumor cells penetrate epithelial basement membrane, gaining access to lymphatics and blood vessels for dissemination*

■ **Host factors**

1. Deficient immune response

❑ *Contributes to development of cancer and metastases*

2. Intact hemostatic system

❏ *Platelets play central role in metastatic process*

❏ *Antiplatelet drugs inhibit experimentally induced cell metastases in mice*

3. Favorable target organ environment

❏ *Tissues may exert growth-promoting or growth-inhibiting effects on cancer cells conducive to neoplastic growth*

Metastatic Sequence

■ **Tumor neovascularization and growth**

1. **Growing tumor establishes its own blood supply through angiogenesis**

2. **As tumor grows, necrotic areas of tumor release chemotactic products that attract host cells and cellular enzymes that help degradate surrounding structures**

■ **Tumor cell invasion of basement membrane and other extracellular matrices**

1. **Local invasion of tissue surrounding tumor can be by single cells or groups of cells**

2. **Invasion begins with destruction of basement membrane of cells of host tissue**

3. **Proteolytic enzymes such as collagenase specific for type IV collagen, plasminogen activator, cathepsins, stromelysin, and heparinase have been implicated in loss of**

basement membrane associated with tumor invasion

■ **Detachment and embolism of tumor cell aggregates**

1. Early movement of tumor cell is by pseudopodia protrusion

2. Random tumor cell motility and dispersion from primary site are regulated by cytokines "autocrine motility factor" and "scatter factor"

3. Direction of tumor cell movement is influenced by host chemo-attractants produced by organ to which tumor cell subsequently travels

4. Tumor cells entering the lymphatic system are transported passively from site of detachment to first draining lymph node where they

   ❑ *Pass through to distant lymph nodes*

   ❑ *Remain in the lymph node to proliferate, die, remain dormant, or enter the bloodstream*

5. Because of numerous connections between lymphatics and vascular system, tumor cells that enter lymphatic system eventually find their way into vascular system

6. In circulatory system, tumor cells face threats such as

   ❑ *Mechanical forces of blood turbulence*
   ❑ *Immune defenses*

7. **Tumor cells form adhesions to other tumor cells or blood cells such as platelets for protection against immune cells**

■ **Arrest**

1. **Tumor cells arrest in capillaries and attach to endothelial cells or vascular basement membrane, or both**

2. **Approximately 50% to 60% of metastatic distribution can be predicted from anatomic route followed by disseminating tumor cell**

3. **In approximately 40% of tumors, distribution of metastases appears**

   ❏ *To be selective*

   ❏ *To depend on growth factors and match between tumor and organ chemotaxis*

■ **Extravasation**

1. **Once tumor cell arrests in capillary bed of target organ**

   ❏ *Degradative enzymes are produced by tumor cells that break down capillary basement membrane*

   ❏ *Tumor cell penetrates through capillary into organ tissue*

■ **Neovascularization and growth of metastasis**

1. **Metastatic tumor grows and proliferates by**

   ❏ *Establishing a blood supply* (angiogenesis)
   ❏ *Restarting metastatic cycle*

Antimetastasis Therapy

■ Prevention of metastasis lies in ability to interrupt one or more steps in metastatic process

■ Many substances that interfere with metastatic process have been studied

1. Razoxane inhibits tumor cell invasion

2. Antiadhesive synthetic peptide Arg-Gly-Asp

3. Monoclonal antibodies prevent tumor cells from binding to and invading basement membrane

4. Heparin and cortisone interfere with tumor neovascularization and coagulation

Clinical Application

■ Clinical challenges of cancer metastasis include

1. Accurate identification of metastatic potential of primary tumor

2. Diagnosis and localization of clinically silent micrometastases at time of initial diagnosis of cancer

3. Complete eradication of all tumor cells in heterogeneous tumor with primary tumor treatment

4. **Selective eradication of metastases during treatment of primary tumor**

5. **Prevention of invasion and metastasis**

Suggested Readings

1. Dujack L: Cancer metastasis. *Semin Oncol Nurs* 8(1):40–50, 1992.

2. Fidler IJ: Critical factors in the biology of human metastasis: Twenty-eighth G. H. A. Clowes Memorial Award Lecture. *Cancer Res* 50:6130–6138, 1990.

3. Groenwald SL: Invasion and metastasis. In Groenwald SL, Frogge MH, Goodman M, Yarbro CH (eds.): *Cancer Nursing: Principles and Practice.* (3rd ed.). Boston: Jones and Bartlett, 1993, pp. 58–69.

4. Killion JJ, Fidler IJ: The biology of tumor metastasis. *Semin Oncol* 16:106–115, 1989.

5. Liotta LA, Kohn E: Cancer invasion and metastases. *JAMA* 263:1123–1126, 1990.

The Immune System and Cancer

Overview

Many immune system components are involved in the body's immunologic response against cancer cells

■ Tumor-associated antigens

1. Located on surfaces of cancer cells

2. Provoke immune reactions in immunocompetent hosts

3. Used clinically as tumor markers for
   ❑ *Diagnostic purposes*
   ❑ *Monitoring prognosis and response to therapy*

4. Detected by
   ❑ *Immunohistologic techniques (tissue)*
   ❑ *Immunochemical techniques (serum)*

5. Types of human tumor-associated antigens include

❏ *Normal tissue antigens associated with differentiation*

☐ Permit definitive identification of tumor tissue of origin

- Human chorionic gonadotropin for placental tumors

- Prostatic acid phosphatase for prostatic cancers

- Immunoglobulin molecules for tumors of B-cell origin

☐ Useful for tumor classification and patient management

❏ *Viral-associated antigens*

☐ Common in many different animal and human tumors

☐ Strong association between development of tumors and viral infections in

- Hepatitis B virus and hepatocellular carcinoma

- Epstein-Barr virus and certain B-cell lymphomas (e.g., Burkitt's lymphoma)

- Human papillomavirus and cervical carcinoma

- Human T-lymphotropic virus type 1 and acute T-cell leukemias

☐ Associations have led to research of vaccines to confer protective antitumor immunity to humans

☐ Existence of tumor-associated viral antigens in humans does not directly implicate that virus in development of a particular malignant disease

- ☐ Genetic mechanism(s) by which viruses induce tumors in humans are poorly understood
- ☐ Effects produced by a virus can be either
  - ■ Direct (as in the case of viral activation of a particular oncogene)
  - ■ Indirect (as in the case of human immunodeficiency virus)
- ❏ *Oncofetal antigens*
  - ☐ Proteins normally present during fetal development that are suppressed to low but still detectable levels in adult
  - ☐ Expressed on tumor tissues and reappear in circulation of patients with malignant disease
  - ☐ Used most frequently in clinical practice to monitor tumor progression and response to treatment
  - ☐ Examples include
    - ■ Carcinoembryonic antigen (CEA) associated with breast, lung, and colorectal tumors
    - ■ Alpha-fetoprotein (AFP) associated primarily with hepatocellular carcinomas and certain germ cell tumors
  - ☐ CEA and AFP may be elevated in cigarette smokers and in nonmalignant diseases including
    - ■ Cirrhosis
    - ■ Obstructive pulmonary diseases

Immunologic Reactions Against Tumor Cells

■ Cells responsible for reactions include

1. T-lymphocytes

❑ *Produce and secrete lymphokines responsible for immune-cell activation, proliferation, and regulation*

❑ *Killer T-lymphocytes mediate tumor cell lysis*

❑ *Suppressor T-lymphocytes are responsible for immune deficiency*

2. Natural killer (NK) cells

❑ *Secrete lymphokines (e.g., interleukin-1 (IL-1), IL-2, tumor necrosis factor-α, interferon-α, and several different hematopoietic colony-stimulating factors)*

❑ *Inhibit tumor growth and regulate antitumor immunity*

3. Lymphokine-activated killer (LAK) cells

❑ *IL-2 increases potency of tumor-killing response of NK cells and T-lymphocytes*

❑ *T-lymphocytes normally require prior exposure to tumor cells to be activated; incubation with IL-2 removes prior exposure requirement*

❑ *Ability of lymphokines to increase tumor-killing capacity of NK cells and T-lymphocytes prompted development of several approaches to immunotherapy*

4. Macrophage-mediated killer cells

❏ *Most important macrophage functions are*
   ☐ Tumor antigen presentation
   ☐ Regulation of other immune-cell types
   ☐ Capacity to destroy tumor cells

❏ *Activation depends on lymphokines, especially interferon-γ*

❏ *Tumor-cell killing does not require prior exposure of macrophage to tumor cell*

❏ *Activated macrophages that are either conjugated to tumor cells or proximal to tumor cells induce state in which there is no cell division or DNA synthesis*

5. Antibody-dependent tumor cell cytotoxicity

❏ *Recognition capabilities of antibodies facilitate tumor cell destruction in collaboration with different immune effector cells*

❏ *NK cells and macrophages can interact with IgG antibody–coated tumor cells, which leads to tumor cell lysis*

How Tumor Cells Evade the Immune System

■ **Tumor cells evade recognition by**

1. Antigenic modulation

❏ *Loss of membrane-associated antigens*

❏ *Modulation of membrane-associated antigenic structures*

2. Modifying expression of membrane-associated structure critical for immune-cell interaction

3. "Blocking factors" such as antibodies hinder sensitized immune effector cells from recognizing and conjugating to tumor cell surfaces

■ Antitumor immunity is suppressed by

1. Secretion of suppressor factors from tumors

2. Hyperactivation of suppressor T-cells and suppressor macrophages during progressive tumor growth

The Importance of the Immune System for Specific Aspects of Neoplasia

■ Role of immune response in carcinogenesis

1. Antitumor immune functions of NK cells, LAK cells, and macrophages during promotion phase of carcinogenesis are most responsible for immune surveillance against developing cancer

2. Progression of malignant tumor may be both positively and negatively influenced by immune reactions

■ **Role of immune response in metastasis**

1. **Inflammatory macrophages activated in response to local tumor growth produce enzymes that**
   ❏ *Participate in destruction of vessel barriers*
   ❏ *Lead to invasion by tumor cells*

2. **Products of activated inflammatory cells facilitate tumor cell embolization with platelets, polymorphonuclear leukocytes, and macrophages: these products help tumor cells survive passage through the circulation**

3. **Metastasizing tumor cells arrested in distant capillary bed are assisted in extravasating through capillary into organ parenchyma by release of degradative enzymes by activated immune cells**

Immunodeficiency in Cancer

■ **Correlates with clinical stage of disease**
■ **Responsible for development of infection**
■ **Associated with a poorer prognosis**

Suggested Readings

1. Applebaum JW: The role of the immune system in the pathogenesis of cancer. *Semin Oncol Nurs* 8(1):51–62, 1992.

2. Braun DP, Groenwald SL: Relation of the immune system to cancer. In Groenwald SL, Frogge MH, Goodman M, Yarbro CH (eds.): *Cancer Nursing: Principles and Practice* (3rd ed.). Boston: Jones and Bartlett, 1993, pp. 70–83.

3. Penn I: Principles of tumor immunity: Immunocompetence and cancer. In Devita VT Jr, Hellman S, Rosenberg SA (eds.): *Biologic Therapy of Cancer.* Philadelphia: Lippincott, 1991, pp. 53–67.

4. Morton DL, Economou J: Cancer immunology and immunotherapy. In Haskell CM (ed.): *Cancer Treatment* (3rd ed.). Philadelphia: WB Saunders, 1990, pp. 102–119.

PART II

Diagnosis and Treatment

■ 6 ■
Diagnostic Evaluation

Overview

■ Major goals are to determine

1. Tissue type
2. Primary site
3. Extent of disease
4. Potential for recurrence

■ Approach depends on

1. Patient's presenting symptoms
2. Patient's clinical status
3. Patient's tolerance of invasive tests
4. Anticipated goal of treatment
5. Biologic characteristics of suspected tumor
6. Availability of diagnostic equipment
7. Third-party payor approval

■ Early detection and treatment are key to survival. The seven warning signals of cancer are

1. Change in bowel or bladder habits
2. Unusual bleeding or discharge
3. Sore that does not heal
4. Obvious change in wart or mole
5. Thickening or lump in breast or elsewhere
6. Nagging cough or hoarseness
7. Indigestion or difficulty in swallowing

Nursing Implications in Diagnostic Evaluation

■ Role of nurse

1. Determine an individual's risk for cancer
2. Facilitate entry into the health care system
3. Provide information on cancer detection and diagnostic procedures
4. Clarify misconceptions
5. Refer patient to appropriate health care providers
6. Provide information and support to reduce stress of evaluation for suspected malignancy
7. Assess for possible complications from procedure
8. Institute appropriate management protocols

Diagnostic Methods

■ Laboratory studies

1. Biochemical analysis of blood and urine

2. Tumor markers

❏ *Produced by tumor*

❏ *Produced by other cells in response to tumor*

❏ *Can be used to detect cancer or monitor response to therapy*

❏ *Most commonly used markers are*
   ☐ Carcinoembryonic antigen
   ☐ Alpha-fetoprotein
   ☐ Human chorionic gonadotropin β-subunit
   ☐ Prostatic acid phosphatase
   ☐ Calcitonin
   ☐ Cancer antigen 125
   ☐ Cancer antigen 153
   ☐ Prostate-specific antigen

■ Tumor imaging

1. Radiographic techniques

2. Nuclear medicine techniques

3. Positron emission tomography

4. Radio-labeled monoclonal antibodies

5. Ultrasonography

6. Magnetic resonance imaging

■ Invasive diagnostic techniques

1. Endoscopy

❏ *Provides direct view by insertion of endoscope into body cavity or opening*

❏ *Permits visual inspection, tissue biopsy, cytologic aspiration, staging of disease, and excision for pathology*

2. Biopsy

❏ *Provides tissue for histologic examination*

❏ *Common techniques include*
- ☐ Needle biopsy
- ☐ Incisional biopsy
- ☐ Excisional biopsy
- ☐ Punch biopsy
- ☐ Bone marrow biopsy

Suggested Readings

1. O'Mary SS: Diagnostic evaluation, classification, and staging. In Groenwald S, Frogge MH, Goodman M, Yarbro CH (eds.): *Cancer Nursing: Principles and Practice* (3rd ed.). Boston: Jones and Bartlett, 1993, 170–193.

2. Lind J: Tumor cell growth and cell kinetics. *Semin Oncol Nurs* 8:3–9, 199–217, 1992.

3. Shellock FG: MRI biologic effects and safety considerations. In Higgins CB, Hricak H, Helms CA (eds.): *Magnetic Resonance Imaging of the Body.* New York: Raven Press, 1992, pp. 233–265.

Principles of Treatment

Classification and Staging

■ Basic terminology

1. *Tumor:* Mass of tissue that may be benign or malignant

2. *Cancer:* Malignant tumor capable of metastasis and invasion

3. *Primary tumor:* Original histologic site of tumorigenesis

4. *Secondary or metastatic tumor:* Resembles primary tumor histologically

5. *Second primary lesion:* New, histologically separate malignant neoplasm in the same patient

6. *Unknown primary:* Biopsy of metastatic site reveals cells that are markedly anaplastic, making it impossible to determine tissue of origin

■ **Tumor classification**

1. Tumors usually retain sufficient characteristics of normal cells to allow recognition of type of tissue from which they were derived

2. Tissue of origin is basis of distinguishing tumors in histogenetic classification system (see Appendix 7–1)

■ **Staging**

1. Method of classifying malignancy by extent of its spread

2. Cancers of similar histologic features and site of origin will invade locally and metastasize in a predictable manner

3. Objectives of staging for solid tumors are to
   ❑ *Aid in treatment planning*
   ❑ *Give prognostic information*
   ❑ *Assist in treatment evaluation*
   ❑ *Facilitate exchange of information*
   ❑ *Compare statistics among treatment centers*

4. **Tumor-Node-Metastasis (TNM) staging system**
   ❑ *Internationally accepted method of staging solid tumors*

   ❑ *Solid tumors are classified by anatomic extent of disease:*
      ☐ *(T):* Extent of primary tumor evaluated on basis of depth of invasion, surface spread, and tumor size

- ☐ *(N):* Absence or presence and extent of regional lymph node metastasis
- ☐ *(M):* Absence or presence of distant metastasis

❏ *Tumors are further classified by*
  - ☐ Clinical extent of disease
  - ☐ Extent of disease after pathologic review
  - ☐ Extent of disease at retreatment
  - ☐ Extent of disease at autopsy

❏ *TNM permits staging groups (I, II, III, and IV) and therapeutic planning*

5. **Other staging systems are**

❏ Clark level: *Melanomas are staged histologically by level of invasion of primary lesion*

❏ Duke's staging system: *Colorectal cancer is classified by depth of invasion and presence of nodal metastasis*

❏ *The* International Federation of Gynecology and Obstetrics *has an accepted staging system for cervical and endometrial cancers*

❏ *Hodgkin's disease and non-Hodgkin's lymphoma are described by the* Ann Arbor classification, *which recognizes disease distribution and symptoms*

❏ *Leukemias are classified according to their predominant cell types, cell maturation, and acute or chronic nature*

■ Grading

1. **Method of classification based on histopathologic characteristics of tissue**

2. Reveals degree of malignancy of tumor cells

3. Compares cellular anaplasia, differentiation, and mitotic activity with normal counterparts

4. American Joint Committee on Cancer recommends the following grading classification

- ❏ *GX: Grade cannot be assessed*
- ❏ *G1: Well differentiated*
- ❏ *G2: Moderately well differentiated*
- ❏ *G3: Poorly differentiated*
- ❏ *G4: Undifferentiated*

◼ **Treatment planning**

1. Involves interdisciplinary decision making based on

- ❏ *Aggressiveness of tumor*
- ❏ *Predictability of spread*
- ❏ *Morbidity and mortality that can be expected from treatment*
- ❏ *Cure rate*
- ❏ *Patient's wishes*

2. Involves entering patients into clinical research trial if one is available

3. Treatment design

- ❏ *May include surgery, chemotherapy, radiation, and/or biotherapy*

❑ *Establish goal of treatment*
  ☐ Cure   ☐ Palliation
  ☐ Control

❑ *Combination therapy is most appropriate if cure is possible*

❑ *More aggressive therapies are appropriate if cure is possible*

❑ *If cure is not possible treatment should not cause more hardship than the cancer*

■ **Assessing response to treatment**

1. Objective criteria are

❑ Complete response (CR): *Complete disappearance of signs and symptoms of disease for at least 1 month*

❑ Partial response (PR): *Fifty percent or more reduction in sum of products of greater and lesser diameters of all measured lesions for at least 1 month, with no new lesions appearing*

❑ Minimal response (MR): *Same as for PR but less than 50% reduction*

❑ Progression: *Twenty-five percent or more increase in sum of all measured lesions, or appearance of new lesions*

❑ Stable disease: *Measurable tumor does not meet criteria for CR, PR, MR, or progression*

2. Subjective criteria include

❑ *Increased feeling of well-being*
❑ *Increased strength*
❑ *Decreased fatigue*

❑ *Improved appetite*
❑ *Weight gain*
❑ *Decreased pain*

Suggested Readings

1. Maxwell MB: Principles of treatment planning. In Groenwald S, Frogge MH, Goodman M, Yarbro CH (eds.) *Cancer Nursing: Principles and Practice* (3rd ed.). Boston: Jones and Bartlett, 1993, pp. 208–221.

2. Beahrs OH, Henson DE, Hutter RVP, et al: *American Joint Committee on Cancer: Manual for Staging of Cancer* (4th ed.). Philadelphia: Lippincott, 1992.

3. Henson DE: Future directions for the American Joint Committee on Cancer. *Cancer* 69(suppl.):1639–1644, 1992.

4. Yarbro JW: Future potential of adjuvant and neoadjuvant therapy. *Semin Oncol* 18:63–69, 1992.

Appendix 7–1

Select Benign and Malignant Neoplasms Listed by Histogenetic Classification

Tissue of Origin	Benign Neoplasm	Malignant Neoplasm
Epithelial (Endodermal)		
Squamous	Squamous cell papilloma	Squamous cell or epidermoid carcinoma
Glandular	Adenoma Papilloma Cystadenoma	Adenocarcinoma Papillary carcinoma Cystadenocarcinoma
Respiratory tract		Bronchogenic carcinoma
Renal epithelium	Renal tubular adenoma	Renal cell carcinoma (hypernephroma)
Urinary tract	Transitional cell papilloma	Transitional cell carcinoma
Placental epithelium	Hydatidiform mole	Choriocarcinoma
Testicular epithelium		Seminoma Embryonal carcinoma
Liver	Liver cell adenoma	Hepatocellular carcinoma (hepatoma)
Biliary tree	Cholangioma	Cholangiocarcinoma
Stomach	Gastric polyp	Gastric carcinoma
Colon	Colonic polyp	Adenocarcinoma of the colon
Mesenchymal (Mesodermal)		
Connective		
Fibrous tissue	Fibroma	Fibrosarcoma
Adipose tissue	Lipoma	Liposarcoma
Cartilage	Chondroma	Chondrosarcoma
Bone	Osteoma	Osteosarcoma

(continued)

Appendix 7–1   (Continued)

Select Benign and Malignant Neoplasms
Listed by Histogenetic Classification

Tissue of Origin	Benign Neoplasm	Malignant Neoplasm
Mesenchymal (Mesodermal) (continued)		
Muscle		
Smooth muscle	Leiomyoma	Leiomyosarcoma
Striated muscle	Rhabdomyoma	Rhabdomyosarcoma
Endothelial		
Blood vessels	Hemangioma	Hemangiosarcoma
Lymphatic vessels	Lymphangioma	Lymphangiosarcoma
Hematopoietic and lymphoreticular		
Hematopoietic cells		Leukemias
Lymphoid tissue		Lymphomas Hodgkin's disease
Plasma cells		Plasmacytoma (multiple myeloma)
Neural (Ectodermal)		
Meninges	Meningioma	Meningeal sarcoma
Glia	Astrocytoma	Glioblastoma multiforme
Nerve cells	Ganglioneuroma	Neuroblastoma Medulloblastoma
Melanocytes	Nevus	Malignant melanoma
Mixed Tissues		
Kidney		Wilms' tumor
Salivary gland	Mixed tumor of salivary gland (pleomorphic adenoma)	Malignant mixed tumor of salivary gland

▪ 8 ▪
Surgical Therapy

Overview

■ Approximately 55% of all individuals with cancer are treated with surgical intervention

■ Of the 40% of individuals treated by surgery alone, one-third are cured

■ Using combinations of surgery, chemotherapy, radiotherapy, and biotherapy, disease-free intervals have been significantly lengthened and survival advantages have been realized

■ Surgery can be used for

1. Cancer prevention
2. Diagnosis
3. Definitive treatment
4. Rehabilitation
5. Palliation

■ Factors influencing treatment decisions

1. Tumor cell kinetics

❏ *Radical surgical procedures used to treat cancer have failed to significantly increase cure rates*

❏ *Recent explosion of knowledge of tumor cell kinetics has helped to identify tumors best treated with surgery*

2. Growth rate

❏ *Slow-growing tumors consisting of cells with prolonged cell cycles lend themselves best to surgical treatment because they are more likely to be confined locally*

3. Invasiveness

❏ *A surgical procedure intended to be curative must resect entire tumor mass and normal tissue surrounding tumor to ensure margin of safety for removal of all cancer cells*

❏ *Less radical procedures are indicated where radical surgery has not proven enhanced results*

4. Metastatic potential

❏ *Initial surgical procedure has better chance for success than subsequent surgery performed for recurrence*

❏ *Knowledge of metastatic patterns of individual tumors is crucial for planning most effective therapy*

❏ *Some tumors metastasize late or not at all and may respond well to aggressive primary surgical resection*

❑ *Some tumors predictably metastasize to local or regional sites; cure may be achieved by removal of primary tumor-bearing organ and adjacent tissues or lymph nodes*

❑ *For tumors known to metastasize early, surgery may not be appropriate, or surgery may be used to remove all visible tumor in preparation for adjuvant systemic therapy or after chemotherapy to resect remaining disease*

5. Tumor location

❑ *Location and extent of tumor determine structural and functional changes after surgery*

❑ *Anticipated changes assist patient and family in weighing benefits and risks of treatment*

❑ *Superficial and encapsulated tumors are more easily resected than those embedded in inaccessible or delicate tissues, or those that have invaded tissues in multiple directions*

6. Physical status

❑ *Preoperative assessment identifies factors that may increase risk of surgical morbidity and mortality; systems to be evaluated are*
  ☐ Respiratory
  ☐ Cardiovascular
  ☐ Nutritional
  ☐ Immunologic
  ☐ Renal
  ☐ Central nervous

❏ *Patient's rehabilitation potential is assessed prior to surgery, and determination is made as to whether individual is capable of handling anticipated physiologic alterations*

7. Quality of life

❏ *Goal of surgical therapy varies with stage of disease*

❏ *Selection of treatment approach takes into consideration quality of individual's life when treatment is complete*

Preventing Cancer Using Surgical Procedures

■ **Surgery may remove nonvital benign tissue that predisposes individual to higher risk of cancer, such as prophylactic removal of breast in women with high risk of breast cancer**

■ **Role of surgery in cancer prevention is limited**

Diagnosing Cancer Using Surgical Techniques

■ **Surgical techniques to biopsy cells or tissue specimens for histologic examination**

1. Selection of biopsy technique depends on possible treatment methods if cancer is diagnosed

2. **Site of biopsy should be removed at surgery, or biopsy should contain tumor in toto**

3. **Biopsy specimen should contain both normal cells and tumor cells for comparison: it should be**

   ❏ *Intact and not crushed or contaminated*

   ❏ *Labeled and preserved properly for complete evaluation*

4. **If multiple biopsy specimens are taken, instruments that may have contacted tumor should not be used for other sites**

5. **Only positive biopsy findings are definitive**

6. **Possible complications of biopsy include**

   ❏ *Pain*   ❏ *Infection*
   ❏ *Bleeding*   ❏ *Dehiscence*
   ❏ *Hematoma*   ❏ *Tumor-cell seeding*

7. **Tell patients when biopsy results will be available and how physician will give results**

■ **Needle biopsy**

1. **Performed in outpatient setting**

2. **Local or topical anesthetic used**

3. **Limitation is possibility that tumor will be missed because of narrow tract of needle**

■ Surgical biopsy (extracted with needle)

1. *Excisional biopsy* is performed on small, accessible tumors to remove entire mass and little or no margin of surrounding normal tissues

2. *Incisional biopsy* is to diagnose large tumors that require major surgery for complete removal

3. *Endoscopy* is for diagnosis of tumors in accessible lumen

Staging Cancer Using Surgical Procedures

■ Exploratory surgical procedures important in defining extent of tumor involvement

■ The American Joint Committee for Cancer Staging and End Results Reporting developed Tumor-Node-Metastasis system for staging many cancers by site (see Chapter 7)

■ Determining stage of disease important in selection of therapy

■ Astute nursing care may alleviate profound anxiety patients experience during diagnostic phase

Surgery for Treatment of Cancer

■ **Surgery aimed at cure**

1. Surgical approach for cure has changed from "more is better" philosophy to consideration of tissue and functional preservation; relies more on adjuvant therapy

2. Type of surgical procedure selected depends on specific tumor cell characteristics and site of involvement

3. Adjuvant or combination therapy with radiotherapy or chemotherapy may be used to improve cure rates and survival

4. Surgery may be used to resect a metastatic lesion if primary tumor is believed to be eradicated and

   ❏ *Metastatic site is solitary*

   ❏ *Patient can undergo surgery without major morbidity*

5. In preoperative period, nurse instructs individual as to what to expect in postoperative recovery and rehabilitation

■ **Surgery aimed at palliation**

1. For palliation of debilitating manifestations of cancer such as pain and obstruction

2. Aimed at controlling cancer and improving quality of life

■ **Surgery for rehabilitation**

1. For cosmetic reasons or to restore function after surgery, such as breast reconstruction, head and neck reconstruction, and skin grafting

■ **Goal is to improve quality of life**

■ **Rehabilitation potential considered before surgery**

Approaches to Care

■ **Special considerations**

1. Patients may donate one or more units of their own blood to bank prior to surgery (*autologous blood donation*)

2. Autologous donation must be completed 42 to 72 hours before surgery

■ **Anxiety and pain control**

1. Patient teaching about pain control begins preoperatively and includes

   ❏ *Expectations of pain and its relief*

   ❏ *Dosing of analgesic medicine*

   ❏ *Use of rating scales to measure pain*

   ❏ *Nonpharmacologic methods to decrease pain and anxiety*

■ Nutrition

1. **Nutritionally debilitated person with cancer is a poor surgical risk**

2. **Prior to surgery, protein calorie malnutrition is reversed, and weight loss prevented**

3. **Patients may receive aggressive preoperative nutritional support to improve nutritional status**

■ Hemostasis

1. **Person with cancer is highly susceptible to postoperative thrombophlebitis**

2. **Early postoperative ambulation is instituted**

3. **The nurse observes patient closely for signs and symptoms of phlebitis**

■ Wound healing

1. **Postoperative complications include**
   - ❏ *Wound dehiscence*

   - ❏ *Infection*

   - ❏ *When surgery is performed on previously irradiated tissue or when chemotherapy is initiated early in the postoperative period, potential complications include*
     - ☐ Postoperative wound dehiscence
     - ☐ Infection
     - ☐ Tissue and bone necrosis

Suggested Readings

1. Kalinowski BH: Surgical therapy. In Groenwald SL, Frogge MH, Goodman M, Yarbro CH (eds.): *Cancer Nursing: Principles and Practice* (3rd ed.). Boston: Jones and Bartlett, 1993, pp. 222–234.

2. Steele G, Cady B: The surgical oncologist as the patient manager. In Steele G, Cady B (eds.): *General Surgical Oncology*. Philadelphia: Saunders, 1992, pp. 18–21.

3. Rosenberg SA: Principles of surgical oncology. In DeVita VT, Hellman S, Rosenberg SA (eds.): *Cancer: Principles and Practice of Oncology* (3rd ed.). Philadelphia: Lippincott, 1989, pp. 236–246.

4. Morton D: Economou JS, Haskell CM, et al: Oncology. In Swartz SI, Shires GT, Spencer FC (eds.): *Principles of Surgery* (5th ed.). New York: McGraw-Hill, 1989, pp. 355–385.

Overview

▪ Radiotherapy may be used

1. As the sole treatment for cancer

2. In combination with surgery or chemotherapy and immunotherapy

▪ The goal may be to

1. Cure (e.g. skin cancer, carcinoma of the cervix, or Hodgkin's disease)

2. Control (e.g. breast cancer, soft-tissue sarcomas, or lung cancer)

3. Palliate (e.g. by relieving pain, preventing pathologic fractures, returning mobility in metastatic bone lesions, and relieving central nervous system (CNS) symptoms caused by brain metastasis or spinal cord compression)

■ Equipment and beams used in radiation are

1. Teletherapy (external radiation)

❏ *Conventional, or orthovoltage, equipment*

- ☐ Produces X rays of varying energies
- ☐ The higher the voltage, the greater the depth of penetration of the x-ray beam
- ☐ Disadvantages include
  - ■ Poor depth of penetration
  - ■ Severe skin reactions because of high dose at skin level
  - ■ Bone necrosis because bone absorbs more than soft tissue

❏ *Megavoltage equipment*

- ☐ Has distinct advantages over orthovoltage
  - ■ Deeper beam penetration
  - ■ More homogeneous absorption of radiation resulting in less bone necrosis
  - ■ Greater skin sparing
- ☐ Equipment includes
  - ■ Van de Graaf generator
  - ■ Cobalt and cesium units
  - ■ Betatron and linear accelerators

2. Brachytherapy

❏ *Use of sealed sources of radioactive material placed within or near tumor*

- ☐ Frequently combined with teletherapy
- ☐ May be used preoperatively and postoperatively
- ☐ Contained in a variety of forms
  - ■ Wires (^{182}Ta)
  - ■ Ribbons or tubes (^{192}Ir)

- Needles (^{137}Cs, ^{226}Ra)
- Grains or seeds (^{198}Au, ^{222}Rn)
- Capsules (^{137}Cs, ^{226}Ra)

☐ Source selected by radiotherapist according to
  - Site to be treated
  - Size of lesion
  - Whether implant is temporary or permanent

☐ Used in treatment of
  - Head and neck lesions (needles, wire, and ribbons)
  - Intra-abdominal and intrathoracic lesions (gold or iodine seeds)
  - Gynecologic tumors

☐ May be
  - Preloaded (radiation present when applicator placed in tissue)
  - Afterloaded (radioactive source added after applicator is in position)

❏ *Brachytherapy is either*
  ☐ Low-dose-rate
  ☐ High-dose-rate (produces same radiobiologic effect in short period of time)

■ Radiobiology

1. Cellular response to radiation

❏ *Direct radiation hit at cellular level occurs when any key molecule within cell (DNA or RNA) is damaged*
  ☐ Unrepaired breaks or alterations lead to mutations and altered cell function or cell death
  ☐ Most effective and lethal injury

❑ *Indirect hit occurs when ionization takes place in medium (mostly water) surrounding molecular structures in cell*

  ☐ Results in free radical that may trigger variety of chemical reactions producing compounds toxic to cell

  ☐ More likely to occur than direct hit

❑ *Radiosensitivity maximum just before and during actual cell division*

❑ *Sensitivity of cells to irradiation is directly proportional to their reproductive activity (radiation most effective during mitosis) and inversely proportional to their degree of differentiation (the more differentiated, the less sensitive to radiation)*

❑ *Cell death from radiation can be immediate or delayed*

❑ *Radiation can inhibit cell from reproducing*

❑ *Other factors that directly affect biologic response to radiation include*

  ☐ *Oxygen effect:* Well-oxygenated tumors have greater response to radiation

  ☐ *Linear energy transfer (LET):* Rate at which energy is lost from different types of radiations while traveling through matter

    ▪ Higher LET has greater probability of interacting with matter and producing more direct hits

  ☐ *Relative biologic effectiveness:* Compares dose of test radiation with dose of standard radiation that produces same biologic response

□ *Fractionation:* Division of total dose of radiation into a number of equal fractions to accomplish

- Repair

  Of intracellular damage by normal cells between daily dose fractions

  Major advantage of fractioning dosages

- Redistribution (within cell cycle)

  With subsequent daily doses of radiation, more and more tumor cells are delayed in cell cycle and reach mitosis as the next dose is given, increasing cell kill

- Repopulation (new growth of normal tissue)

  Takes place some time during fractionated treatment course

  Fractionation favors normal tissue while still eradicating tumor

- Reoxygenation

  Oxygenated cells are more radiosensitive

  Fractionating dose allows time between treatments for tumors to reoxygenate

■ Chemical and thermal modifiers of radiation

1. Radiosensitizers

❏ *Increase radiosensitivity of tumor cells*
❏ *Achieve greater cell kill*
❏ *Prevent repair of cellular radiation damage*
❏ *Side effects include*

□ Neurotoxicity

□ CNS symptoms of somnolence, confusion, and transient coma

□ Dose-related nausea and vomiting

❏ *Results are disappointing because of severe toxicity and lack of significant efficacy*

2. Radioprotectors

❏ *Protect aerated (nontumor) cells while having limited effect on hypoxic (tumor) cells*

❏ *Increase therapeutic ratio by promoting repair of irradiated normal tissues*

❏ *Nursing responsibilities include*
  ☐ Providing patient and family education
  ☐ Participating in obtaining informed consent
  ☐ Administering investigational agents
  ☐ Timing and coordinating drug administration with radiotherapy treatment
  ☐ Observing and documenting expected and previously unreported effects and side effects
  ☐ Managing side effects, including developing interventions for those newly observed

3. Hyperthermia

❏ *Heat is cytotoxic to cancer cells*

❏ *Hyperthermia combined with radiotherapy produces greater effect than either modality alone*

❏ *Parameters that may influence tumor response to combined hyperthermia and radiation therapy include*
  ☐ Tumor size
  ☐ Histologic findings
  ☐ Disease site
  ☐ Total dose of radiation and dose per fraction

  - ☐ Thermal dose
  - ☐ Total and weekly number of hyperthermia sessions
  - ☐ Sequencing of hyperthermia and radiation

❏ *Hyperthermia is achieved by*
  - ☐ Immersion of local area in heated bath
  - ☐ Ultrasound
  - ☐ Microwaves
  - ☐ Interstitial implants
  - ☐ Perfusion techniques

❏ *Side effects include*
  - ☐ Local skin reaction
  - ☐ Pain
  - ☐ Fever
  - ☐ Gastrointestinal effects
  - ☐ Cardiac arrhythmias
  - ☐ Late effects such as necrosis and ulceration; these are generally not severe enough to discontinue use

❏ *Nursing responsibilities*
  - ☐ Pretreatment evaluation phase
    - ▪ Assess for
      Suitability for treatment
      Ability to tolerate treatment
      Cardiac and neurologic status
      Presence of metal objects
    - ▪ Provide thorough patient and family education
  - ☐ Treatment phase
    - ▪ Monitor vital signs
    - ▪ Prepare patient's gastrointestinal tract

- Administer sedation
- Assist during surgical placement of thermometry probes
- Position patient for comfort and access to applicator probes
- Monitor patient throughout treatment
- Provide physical and emotional support
□ Post-treatment phase
    - Clean and dress cannula sites
    - Observe and document thermal changes at treatment site
    - Provide discharge instructions
    - Manage subsequent local reaction

Simulation

■ **Localizes tumor**

■ **Defines volume to be treated**

■ **Determines field of treatment**

1. **Radiation therapist duplicates markings on patient's skin by tattooing (dropping India ink on patient's skin and introducing ink into skin using needle)**

2. **Patient is immobilized with headrests, armboards, handgrips**

3. **Blocks to protect vital body organs and tissues are secured to plastic tray placed at head of treatment machine between beam and person being treated**

4. **Careful explanation about purpose of simulation and equipment allays patient's anxiety**

Radiation Side Effects

■ **Integumentary system**

1. **Skin is irradiated when any site within body is treated**

2. **Skin of exit portal may also be affected**

3. **Skin reactions may range from erythema to dry and then moist desquamation**

4. **Healing may be slow, but is usually complete, leaving minimal residual damage except for change in pigmentation**

5. **Fibrosis, atrophy, ulceration, necrosis, and skin cancer may occur after high doses, but are uncommon with modern equipment**

6. **Skin in warm, moist areas such as groin, gluteal fold, axilla, and under breast exhibits greater and often earlier reaction to radiation**

7. **Radiation of hair follicles and sweat and sebaceous glands results in loss of hair and decreased activity of glands; both generally return to normal after therapy**

■ Hematopoietic system

1. **If large areas of red bone marrow are irradiated (ilia, vertebrae, ribs, metaphyses of long bones, skull, and sternum), the number of circulating mature blood cells decreases because production is suppressed**

   ❏ *Erythroblasts (red blood cell precursors) are damaged, causing anemia, but recovery is rapid and anemia is transient*

   ❏ *Myeloblasts (white blood cell precursors) are suppressed at same rate as erythroblasts, but rate of recovery is much slower*

   ❏ *Megakaryocytes (platelet precursors) are affected 1 to 2 weeks after exposure and take longest time to recover (2–6 weeks)*

■ Gastrointestinal system

1. **Oral cavity**

   ❏ *Oral mucous membrane may develop a confluent mucositis*

      □ Occurs especially on soft palate and floor of mouth

      □ Occurs during third and fourth weeks of therapy at usual dose rate

   ❏ *Salivary function is altered from damage to serous and mucous acini*

   ❏ *Saliva becomes viscous after moderate doses*

❏ *Higher doses lead to atrophy of salivary glands with greatly diminished saliva and increased acidity*

　□ May be permanent

　□ May lead to radiation caries and infection

❏ *Alterations in taste occur early in treatment but are rarely permanent, depending on dose*

2. Esophagus and stomach

❏ *Gastric secretions of mucus, pepsin, and hydrochloric acid are reduced and may be accompanied by nausea, dyspepsia, and pyloric spasm*

❏ *Gastritis and esophagitis occur with moderate to high doses and produce dysphagia, anorexia, and sometimes nausea and vomiting*

❏ *Late changes may include atrophy, ulcerations, and fibrosis*

3. Small intestine

❏ *Most sensitive area of the gastrointestinal tract*

❏ *Radiation reaction characterized by shortening of villi and loss of absorptive surface*

❏ *Prolonged and severe reactions may cause major nutritional consequences*

❏ *Late changes following high doses of radiation include fibrosis, ulceration, necrosis, and hemorrhage*

❏ *Intestinal obstruction may occur*

❏ *Most common symptoms are anorexia, nausea, diarrhea, and cramping*

4. Colon and rectum

❑ *Effect is similar to that of small intestine*

❑ *Tenesmus may occur when anal sphincter is irradiated*

5. Liver

❑ *Greatest damage to liver is vascular injury*

❑ *Early changes detectable only by liver function test*

❑ *Radiation hepatitis is possible consequence of high doses*

■ **Respiratory system**

1. **Hoarseness due to laryngeal mucous membrane congestion sometimes occurs**

2. **Radiation pneumonitis may be a transient response to moderate doses**

3. **Later changes are fibrosis in lung tissue and thickening of pleura**

■ **Reproductive system**

1. **Cervix and uterine body are radioresistant**

2. **Vaginal mucous membrane responds with mucositis and inflammation**

3. **Vaginal stenosis may be result of brachytherapy**

4. **Radiation to ovaries may produce temporary or permanent sterility, depending on age of person being treated and radiation dose**

5. **Hormonal changes and early menopause may occur after radiation of ovaries**

6. Genetic damage may occur after radiation of gonads in both males and females

7. Radiation to male testes damages and prevents maturation of sperm

8. Sterility may be permanent even in low doses

■ Urinary system

1. Radiation-induced cystitis and urethritis are early and transient effects

2. In high doses nephritis may occur, which may result in renal failure and death

3. Kidneys are protected when abdomen is irradiated

■ Cardiovascular system

1. Damage to vasculature of an organ or tissue can be primary reason for its radioresponsiveness

2. Blood vessels may become occluded when excessive cell production takes place during repair and regeneration in response to radiation injury

3. Thrombosis may be induced by the thickening that occurs during regenerative activity, further occluding vessels

4. Late changes are telangiectasia, petechiae, and sclerosis

5. Heart muscle is relatively radioresistant, although pericarditis may occur

■ Nervous system

1. Brain, spinal cord, and peripheral nerves are relatively radioresistant; damage relates to vascular insufficiency

2. Higher doses may produce transient symptoms in CNS

3. Lhermitte's sign may occur
   ❑ *Follows irradiation to cervical cord*
   ❑ *Characterized by paresthesia in form of shocklike sensations that radiate down back and extremities when neck is bent forward*

4. Myelopathy usually is transient, but at higher doses may lead to paralysis or paresis

5. Radiation of large volumes of spinal cord produces transverse myelitis

6. Radiation to neurons in olfactory, gustatory, and retinal receptors alters or destroys function of sense organ

7. Preexistence of diabetes, hypertension, and arteriosclerosis enhances radiation effects on nervous tissue

■ Skeletal system

1. Mature bone and cartilage are radioresistant

2. Late avascular necrosis
   ❑ *Is rare, but can occur after high doses*
   ❑ *Causes pain and possible pathologic fracture*

3. Radiation has severe effect on growing bone and cartilage, causing deformities and stunting growth

Systemic Effects of Radiation

■ Patients may experience systemic effects of radiation including

1. Nausea

2. Anorexia

3. Malaise resulting from release of toxic waste products into bloodstream from tumor destruction

Nursing Care of the Patient Receiving Radiotherapy

■ General

1. Develop nursing care plan

2. Assist patient in coping with diagnosis

3. Teach patient what to expect

4. Teach patient about expected side effects

5. Assist in arranging transportation for outpatients

6. Prepare patient for

- ❏ *What equipment will look like*
- ❏ *Where radiation department is located*

7. Coordinate complex treatment schedules

■ For fatigue

1. May be pronounced during and after course of radiation treatment

2. Potential causes include

- ❏ *Recent surgery*
- ❏ *Prior or concurrent chemotherapy*
- ❏ *Pain*
- ❏ *Malnourishment*
- ❏ *Medications*
- ❏ *Frequency of treatment visits*
- ❏ *Maintaining usual lifestyle*
- ❏ *Tumor burden*
- ❏ *Anemia*
- ❏ *Respiratory compromise*

3. Extra rest and reduction in normal activity level may be necessary

■ For mucositis

1. Tell patient to avoid irritants such as

- ❏ *Alcohol*
- ❏ *Tobacco*
- ❏ *Spicy or acidic foods*
- ❏ *Very hot or very cold foods and drinks*
- ❏ *Commercial mouthwash products*

2. Tell patient to gargle

- ❏ *As often as every 3 to 4 hours and especially before bed*

❏ *With solution of 1 ounce of diphenhydramine hydrochloride (Benadryl) elixir diluted in 1 quart of water*

3. **Outpatients can irrigate mouth with this solution sprayed into the mouth from an air-powered spray apparatus**
   ❏ *Loosens retained food particles*
   ❏ *Breaks up mucus and soothes mucosa*

4. **Inpatients can modify technique by using disposable irrigation bag hung from pole to deliver spray of solution**

5. **Do not dislodge plaque-like formations of mucositis**

6. **Agents that coat and soothe oral mucosa, such as Maalox, are sometimes used**

7. **Lidocaine hydrochloride 2% viscous solution may provide some relief from discomfort, but anesthetic effect, especially to the tongue, is objectionable to some**

▦ **For xerostomia**

1. **Frequently accompanied by alterations in taste**

2. **Little can be done to relieve this symptom**

3. **Best method is frequent sips of water**

4. **Frequent mouth care provides relief for thick and viscous saliva**

5. **When inflammation has subsided, some individuals benefit from use of saliva substitute for 2- to 4-hour periods**

   ❏ *May assist individuals who otherwise awaken during night because of dry mouth*

   ❏ *Packaged in small container carried easily in pocket or purse*

   ❏ *Formula is*

Cologel	98.2 ml
Glycerin	110.0 ml
Saline	1000.0 ml

   ❏ *Solution is mixed well and refrigerated*

   ❏ *Patient uses 1 to 2 teaspoons every 3 or 4 hours, swishing in mouth and swallowing*

■ **For radiation caries**

1. **Potential late effect of radiation to mouth and oropharynx**

2. **Can be greatly reduced or avoided by proper care before, during, and after course of treatment**

3. **Before therapy, thorough dental examination and prophylaxis should be carried out**

4. **For poor dentition, full mouth extraction is treatment of choice**

5. **If teeth are in good repair, vigorous preventive program is begun**

   ❏ *Daily diphenhydramine hydrochloride mouth spray for cleansing effect*

❑ *Followed by 5-minute application of fluoride gel*

6. **Patient should brush teeth with soft-bristled brush several times daily**

■ **For esophagitis and dysphagia**

1. **Occurs when radiation is directed to mediastinum**

2. **Transient**

3. **First signs are difficulty swallowing solids, progressing to esophagitis, with painful swallowing**

4. **Administer following mixture to provide relief**

   Mylanta: 450 ml (three 5-oz bottles)

   Lidocaine hydrochloride viscous 2%: 100 ml

   Diphenhydramine hydrochloride elixir: 60 ml

   Shake well and refrigerate. Dosage: 1 to 2 tablespoons 15 minutes before meals and at bedtime

5. **In place of regular meals encourage high-calorie, high-protein, high-carbohydrate liquids and soft, bland foods (e.g., eggnog, milk shakes, "instant" liquid meals and commercially prepared liquid supplements, and blenderized foods)**

■ **For nausea and vomiting**

1. **Not common, but occur when treatment is directed to whole abdomen or portions of it, large pelvic fields, hypochondrium, epigastrium, or para-aortic areas**

2. Occurs from 1 to 3 hours after treatment

3. Delay intake of full meal until 3 or 4 hours after treatment

■ **For diarrhea**

1. Not an expected side effect

2. Occurs if areas of abdomen and pelvis are treated with higher doses of radiation

3. Ranges from increased number of bowel movements to loose, watery stools and intestinal cramping

4. Occasionally, treatment interrupted to allow bowel to recover, especially in elderly or debilitated individuals

5. Intravenous fluids for short-term replacement may be needed

6. Low-residue diet and loperamide hydrochloride are usually sufficient to control diarrhea

■ **For tenesmus, cystitis, and urethritis**

1. Infrequent

2. Occur in some individuals receiving pelvic irradiation

❏ *Tenesmus*
   ☐ Produces persistent sensation of need to evacuate bowel or bladder
   ☐ Relief may be obtained from gastrointestinal and urinary antispasmodics and anticholinergic preparations
   ☐ May persist until treatment has ended

❏ *Cystitis and urethritis*
  □ Result from radiation to bladder
  □ If clean-catch urine specimen positive, antibiotic therapy instituted
  □ Usually no infection is found
  □ Treatment consists of urinary antiseptics and antispasmodics for symptomatic relief
  □ High fluid intake is encouraged
  □ Sitz baths contraindicated if perineal area is being irradiated

■ **For alopecia**

1. **Occurs during treatment of whole brain**

2. **Follows typical pattern**
  ❏ *First patient notices excessive amounts of hair in brush or comb, and gradual thinning of hair; this continues about 2 or 3 weeks*
  ❏ *Suddenly, most of hair comes out—patient awakens to find remainder of hair on pillow*
    □ Prepare patient with wig or attractive scarf or hat
    □ Occasionally hair loss occurs regionally or in patches
      ■ Encourage patient to grow hair longer to cover spot

3. **Care of hair and scalp during radiation treatment includes**
  ❏ *Gentle brushing or combing*
  ❏ *Infrequent shampooing*
  ❏ *Permanent waves and hair coloring are contraindicated*

4. **Top of patient's head should be protected from sunburn with a cap**

5. **Forehead, ears, and neck may be more sensitive to sun**

■ **For skin reactions**

1. **Response of skin varies from mild erythema to moist desquamation that leaves raw surface similar to second-degree burn**

2. **Healing and cosmesis usually are satisfactory**

3. **Some individuals exhibit permanent tanning effect in treatment area, with no change in texture of skin**

4. **Others have**
   - ❏ *Fibrosclerotic changes in subcutaneous structures*
   - ❏ *Skin is smooth, taut, and shiny*
   - ❏ *Telangiectasia may be evident*

5. **Skin reactions in groin, perineum, buttocks, inframammary folds, and axillae will be more severe because of warmth and moisture in these areas**

6. **Skin care measures during treatment and until skin reaction has disappeared include**
   - ❏ *Keeping skin dry*
   - ❏ *Avoiding powders, lotions, creams, alcohol, and deodorants*
   - ❏ *Wearing loose-fitting garments*

❏ *Not applying tape to treatment site when dressings are applied*

❏ *Shaving with electric razor only and avoiding preshaves or aftershaves*

❏ *Protecting skin from exposure to direct sunlight, chlorinated swimming pools, and temperature extremes*

7. **Treatment of skin reactions includes**

❏ *Using light dusting of cornstarch for pruritus from erythema and dry desquamation*

❏ *For moist desquamation and denuded areas, using thin layer of A & D ointment followed by nonstick dressing*

8. **Treatment may be required on exit portal as well as marked area**

■ **For bone marrow depression**

1. **Occurs when large areas of active bone marrow are irradiated (especially pelvis or spine in adult)**

2. **Weekly or two to three times weekly blood counts are done on all individuals receiving radiotherapy**

3. **Transfusions of whole blood, platelets, or other components may be necessary for patient with dangerously low blood counts**

4. **Treatment may have to be adjusted or suspended**

5. **Nurse observes for signs and symptoms of bleeding, anemia, and infection**

6. **Patients and families taught what to look for and to report whenever symptoms occur**

■ **For uncommon side effects**

1. **Transient myelitis**

   ❏ *Occurs when lymph nodes in cervical region are radiated*

   ❏ *Lhermitte's sign (a shocklike sensation radiating down back and over extremities when flexing neck) may occur after a 2- to 3-week latent period after treatment ends*

   ❏ *Symptoms improve gradually or spontaneously with no residual effect*

2. **Parotitis**

   ❏ *Painful swelling and inflammation of parotid glands*

   ❏ *Occurs in individual receiving radiation to maxillomandibular area*

   ❏ *Onset is sudden and follows first two or three treatments*

   ❏ *Symptoms subside quickly and require no treatment*

3. **Visual and olfactory disturbances**

   ❏ *Occur during radiation to pituitary area*

   ❏ *Manifest in person seeing lights or smelling something burning after several treatments*

❑ *May relate to irritation of optic nerve and olfactory bulb*

❑ *Reassurance and explanation are best means of handling*

4. **Radiation recall**

❑ *Can occur in a previously irradiated site that exhibited mucositis or erythema*

❑ *Occurs in response to systemic administration of certain chemotherapeutic agents several months to a year or more after radiation received*

❑ *Person develops intraoral mucositis or skin reaction in exact pattern corresponding to previously treated radiation portal*

❑ *Treatment is symptomatic*

Nursing Care of the Patient with a Radioactive Source

■ **Specific safety precautions are to be observed by patients receiving brachytherapy**

■ **To design an appropriate care regimen and safety precautions, the nurse must know the answers to the following**

1. **What is the source being used?**

2. **What is the half-life of that source?**

3. **What is the type of emission (alpha, beta, gamma)?**

4. How much radioisotope is being used?

5. What method of administration or application is being used?

6. Is the source metabolized? Absorbed? Neither?

■ Three major factors are considered in developing safety plans:

1. *Time:* Exposure to radiation is directly proportional to time spent within a specific distance from source

2. *Distance:* Amount of radiation reaching a given area decreases as distance increases

3. *Shield:* Sheet of absorbing material placed between radiation source and detector; amount of radiation reaching detector decreases, depending on energy of radiation and nature and thickness of absorbing material

   ❏ *Portable radiation shields are available*

   ❏ *Useful for doing tasks within room, but not for direct care*

■ Patient education includes

1. Description of procedure

2. Preparation for potential change in appearance (needle implants in facial area)

3. Knowledge of anticipated pain or discomfort and measures available for relief

4. Knowledge of potential short-term and long-term side effects and complications

5. **Restrictions on activity while radioactive sources are in place**

6. **Visiting restrictions**

7. **Radiation precautions observed by hospital personnel**

8. **Preparation for isolation by planning suitable activities such as reading, handiwork, and television**

Suggested Readings

1. Hilderley LJ: Radiotherapy. In Groenwald SL, Frogge MH, Goodman M, Yarbro CH: *Cancer Nursing: Principles and Practice* (3rd ed.). Boston: Jones and Bartlett, 1993, pp. 235–269.

2. Hassey-Dow K, Hilderley L (eds.): *Nursing Care in Radiation Oncology.* Philadelphia: WB Saunders, 1992.

3. Sitton E: Early and late radiation-induced skin alterations. Part I: Mechanisms of skin changes. *Oncol Nurs Forum* 19:801–807, 1992.

4. Sitton E: Early and late radiation-induced skin alterations. Part II: Nursing care of irradiated skin. *Oncol Nurs Forum* 19:907–912, 1992.

Chemotherapy

Principles of Therapy

■ **Factors influencing chemotherapy effectiveness**

1. Biologic characteristics of tumors

❏ Growth rate: *Actively dividing cells are most sensitive to chemotherapy*

❏ Growth fraction: *Number of cells dividing at one time is small*

❏ Tumor cell heterogeneity: *Tumor cells vary in their sensitivity to chemotherapy*

❏ Tumor burden: *The larger the tumor burden, the more likely it is that resistant cells will emerge*

❏ Genetic instability: *Tumor cells can mutate, becoming resistant over time to chemotherapy*

2. Host characteristics include the patient's

❏ *Nutritional status*

❑ *Level of immune function*

❑ *Physical and psychologic tolerance to treatment*

❑ *Response to supportive therapies*

3. **Response to a specific drug or drug regimen is related to**

❑ *Dose*
❑ *Schedule of adminstration*
❑ *Toxicity of drug*
❑ *Route of administration*
❑ *Drug resistance*

Therapeutic Strategies

■ Combination chemotherapy

1. **Use of multiple agents with different actions may**

❑ *Provide maximal cell kill for resistant cells*

❑ *Minimize development of resistant cells*

❑ *Provide maximum cell kill with tolerable toxicity*

■ Scheduling and drug sequencing

1. **Measures to prevent acquired drug resistance include**

❑ *Administering intermittent high doses of drugs*

❑ *Alternating noncross-resistant chemotherapy regimens*

❑ *Minimizing interval between treatments to coincide with recovery of normal cells*

❑ *Maintaining optimum duration of therapy without dose reductions or treatment delays*

■ Dose

1. **Dose reductions and treatment delays most often account for suboptimal response to chemotherapy**

2. **Critical aspects of dosing**

   ❑ Dose size *refers to amount of drug delivered to patient when corrected for pharmacologic variables such as creatinine clearance and weight*

   ❑ Total dose *is sum of all doses of drug for an individual*

   ❑ Dose rate *or dose intensity is amount of drug delivered per unit of time (mg/m^2/week)*

■ *Adjuvant chemotherapy:* **Administration of chemotherapy as a strategy to increase cure rates in individuals with microscopic disease**

■ *Modifying agents:* **Drugs that are used to enhance efficacy of an antineoplastic agent**

■ Reversing multidrug resistance

1. *Multidrug resistance* **occurs when exposure to a single drug is followed by cross-resistance to other drugs**

2. **Major strategies to overcome multidrug resistance include**

❑ *Increasing intracellular drug concentration using high doses of drugs*

❑ *Alternating noncross-resistant chemotherapy regimens*

❑ *Using monoclonal antibodies*

❑ *Maintaining intracellular drug concentration by enhancing the membrane permeability and drug efflux pump*

Clinical Trials

■ *Clinical trial* **is a scientific study designed to answer important clinical and biologic questions**

■ **Conducted according to a written guideline for the study (protocol)**

■ **Provides mechanism to test effectiveness of new therapies**

■ **Clinical trials are categorized as**

1. **Phase I studies**

❑ *Testing done in patients who may benefit from the drugs and for whom there is no treatment known to be superior*

❑ *Goals of phase I study are to*
  ☐ Evaluate acute toxicities
  ☐ Establish maximum tolerated dose
  ☐ Analyze pharmacologic data

2. Phase II studies

❏ *Goals of phase II study are to*
  ☐ Determine tumor activity
  ☐ Design administration techniques
  ☐ Identify precautions and toxicity
  ☐ Determine dose modifications
  ☐ Identify need for supportive care

3. Phase III studies

❏ *Goals of phase III study are to*
  ☐ Compare drug(s) to standard
  ☐ Evaluate response and duration of response
  ☐ Evaluate toxicity and quality-of-life issues

4. Phase IV studies

❏ *Goals of phase IV study are to*
  ☐ Determine new ways to use drug
  ☐ Determine effect of drug in adjuvant therapy

Classification of Antineoplastic Agents

■ **Alkylating agents**

1. Cell cycle nonspecific

2. Mechanism of action is cross-linking strands of DNA

3. Examples include

❏ *Nitrogen mustard*   ❏ *Carboplatin*
❏ *Cyclophosphamide*   ❏ *Ifosfamide*
❏ *Melphalan*   ❏ *Dacarbazine*
❏ *Lomustine*

■ Antitumor antibiotics

1. **Cell cycle nonspecific**

2. **Interfere with DNA function**

3. **Examples include**

   - ❏ *Bleomycin*
   - ❏ *Mitomycin C*
   - ❏ *Daunorubicin*
   - ❏ *Doxorubicin*
   - ❏ *Mitoxantrone*

■ Plant alkaloids

1. **Topoisomerase inhibitors**

2. **Interfere with mitotic activity**

3. **Cell cycle specific**

4. **Examples include**

   - ❏ *Vincristine*
   - ❏ *Vinblastine*
   - ❏ *Etoposide*
   - ❏ *Teniposide*
   - ❏ *Vindesine*

■ Taxanes

1. **Cell cycle specific**

2. **Promote microtubule assembly**

3. **Examples include**

   - ❏ *Taxol*
   - ❏ *Taxotere*

■ Antimetabolites

1. **Cell cycle specific**

2. **Interfere with DNA synthesis**

3. Examples include

- ❏ *Methotrexate*
- ❏ *5 Fluorouracil*
- ❏ *Mercaptopurine*
- ❏ *Cytarabine*

Chemotherapy Administration

■ **Professional qualifications**

1. **Current licensure as registered nurse**

2. **Certification in CPR**

3. **Intravenous therapy skills**

4. **Educational preparation and demonstration of knowledge in all areas related to antineoplastic drugs**

5. **Drug administration skills**

6. **Policies and procedures to govern nursing actions include**

- ❏ *Chemotherapy drug preparation and handling guidelines that comply with Occupational Safety and Health Administration guidelines*

- ❏ *Chemotherapy administration procedures*

- ❏ *Vesicant management*

- ❏ *Management of allergic reactions*

- ❏ *Safe drug handling and disposal*

- ❏ *Patient and family education*

   ❑ *Management of vascular access devices (VADs)*

   ❑ *Documentation methods*

   ❑ *Outcome standards*

   ❑ *Oncology quality-improvement process*

■ **Handling cytotoxic drugs**

1. **All chemotherapy drugs are prepared under a class II biologic safety hood**

2. **Personal protective equipment (PPE) is worn during handling of chemotherapy**

3. **Direct exposure to cytotoxic drugs can occur during admixture, administration, or handling; specifically by inhalation, ingestion, or absorption**

4. **Drugs are known to be mutagenic, teratogenic, and carcinogenic**

■ **Nurse's role in patient and family education about cancer and its treatment**

1. **Identify specific learning needs related to chemotherapy**

2. **Prepare teaching aids such as written materials, calendar, video, teaching guides**

3. **Describe various sensations patient will experience during treatment; e.g., stuffy nose, lightheadedness, dizziness**

4. **Describe specific side effects and measures to prevent these complications**

5. **Teach patients self-care measures and give clear instructions on how to report symptoms**

6. **Ensure that informed consent has been obtained**

7. **Document teaching in patient's medical record and describe method of follow-up**

▪ Administration principles

1. **Most patients receive chemotherapy on an outpatient basis**

2. **To administer an antineoplastic drug**

   ❑ *Verify patient's identity*

   ❑ *Check and double-check drug order*

   ❑ *Calculate body surface area to confirm dosage*

   ❑ *Ensure informed consent*

   ❑ *Evaluate laboratory results*

   ❑ *Locate extravasation kit or supplies if giving vesicant*

   ❑ *Wash your hands, don gloves and other PPE*

   ❑ *Select equipment and site for venipuncture*

   ❑ *Use an appropriate sterile technique for venous access*

   ❑ *Tape needle securely, without obstructing site*

   ❑ *Test vein with at least 5 to 8 cc of normal saline*

   ❑ *Administer chemotherapy with even steady pressure*

❑ *Check for blood return every couple of cubic centimeters of drug given*

❑ *Flush between each drug to avoid incompatibilities*

❑ *When the injection or infusion is complete, dispose of all equipment according to policies and procedures of your institution*

❑ *Arrange for follow-up care*

❑ *Document procedure in patient's medical record*

■ **Vesicant extravasation**

1. **Vesicant drugs can cause tissue necrosis if they infiltrate out of blood vessel and into soft tissue**

2. **Vesicant drugs include**

❑ *Dactinomycin*	❑ *Vinblastine*
❑ *Daunomycin*	❑ *Nitrogen mustard*
❑ *Doxorubicin*	❑ *Idarubicin*
❑ *Mitomycin-C*	❑ *Teniposide*
❑ *Vincristine*	

3. **Extravasation of vesicant can result in physical deformity or functional deficit**

4. **Measures to minimize risk of extravasation**

❑ *Identify patients at risk*

☐ Patients who are unable to communicate clearly

☐ Elderly, confused, debilitated patients with frail, fragile veins

❏ *Avoid infusing vesicants over joints, bony prominences, tendons, or antecubital fossa*

❏ *Avoid giving vesicant drugs in areas where venous or lymphatic circulation is poor*

❏ *Give vesicant agent before other agents*

❏ *If vesicant is ordered as an infusion, it is given only through central line*

❏ *Have on hand extravasation kit and all materials necessary to manage extravasation*

5. **Symptoms of extravasation include**
   - ❏ *Swelling at injection site*
   - ❏ *Stinging, burning, or pain at injection site*
   - ❏ *Redness*
   - ❏ *Lack of blood return*

6. **If extravasation is suspected, stop infusion and follow official policy and procedure for extravasation**

■ **Irritant drugs**

1. **Irritant drugs cause localized irritation, even burning, but no tissue necrosis if infiltrated. Examples include**

❏ *Examples include*	❏ *Etoposide*
❏ *Carmustine*	❏ *Plicamycin*
❏ *Dacarbazine*	❏ *Streptozocin*

■ **Routes of drug administration**

1. Topical   4. Subcutaneous

2. Oral   5. Intravenous

3. Intramuscular   6. Intrathecal

7. Intraperitoneal   9. Intravesical

8. Intrapleural

■ **Vascular access devices (VAD)**

1. Nontunnelled central venous catheters

❏ *Indicated for short-term use*
❏ *Multilumen catheter permits polydrug therapy*
❏ *Easily removed*
❏ *Sterile technique used during care*

2. Tunnelled central venous catheters

❏ *Indicated for frequent IV access*

❏ *Cuff surrounds catheter, permitting fibrous ingrowth*

❏ *Require sterile site care with dressings until formation of granulation tissue*

❏ *Require every other day or weekly flushing (Groshong catheter)*

❏ *Flush with 3 to 5 cc of heparinized saline (10–100 units/cc)*

❏ *Avoid intraluminal mixing of potentially incompatible drugs by flushing with saline between each drug*

3. Implantable ports

❏ *Completely implanted under skin*

❏ *Permit access to venous or arterial system, or peritoneal, pleural, or epidural space*

❏ *Accessed by noncoring needle*

4. Complication management

❏ *Intraluminal catheter occlusion*

 ☐ Complication arises from
  - Blood clot within catheter
  - Crystallization or precipitate
  - Improper needle placement in port

 ☐ Prevention and management
  - Maintain positive pressure during flush
  - Avoid excessive manipulation of catheter
  - Vigorously flush with 20 cc saline after blood draw
  - Flush between each drug to prevent incompatibility
  - Flush every 8 to 12 hours when giving total parenteral nutrition (TPN) or lipids
  - Urokinase may be used if blood clot is suspected

❏ *Extraluminal catheter occlusion*

 ☐ Complication arises from
  - Fibrin sheath formation
  - Thrombosis
  - Catheter position
  - Pinch-off syndrome

 ☐ Prevention and management
  - Vigorously flush to prevent fibrin sheath formation
  - Lyse fibrin sheath with urokinase with dwell time of 24 hours
  - Low-dose warfarin may prevent or decrease incidence of thrombus formation
  - Anticoagulants may be necessary to treat venous thrombosis

❏ *Infection*
  ☐ Manifestations
    ▪ Most common in patients with neutropenia, multilumen catheters, and those receiving TPN
    ▪ Local skin infections common
    ▪ Symptoms include redness, warmth, discomfort, exudate and fever
  ☐ Prevention and management
    ▪ Provide meticulous catheter care
    ▪ Culture area
    ▪ Increase frequency of catheter care
    ▪ Administer appropriate antibiotics
    ▪ Take blood cultures (intraluminal and peripheral)

Management of Chemotherapy Toxicities

■ **Acute and long-term toxicities are often function of effect of drugs on rapidly dividing cells**

■ **Incidence and severity of toxicities are related to**

1. **Drug dosage**
2. **Administration schedule**
3. **Specific mechanism of action**

4. Concomitant illness

5. Measures employed to prevent or minimize toxicities

■ **Pretreatment evaluation: Vigorous treatment course will not be tolerated in**

1. Patients in weak physical condition

2. Patients with poor nutritional status

3. Heavily pretreated patients who may lack marrow reserve, placing them at higher risk for infection, bleeding, or anemia

4. Individuals who are unable or unwilling to care for self

5. Patients with preexisting hepatic or renal dysfunction which can alter absorption, distribution, metabolism, and excretion of drugs

6. Patients with hypovolemia and dehydration from nausea, vomiting, or diarrhea, which may increase risk of acute renal failure

7. Patients with a concomitant illness that affects individual's ability to metabolize drug or to care for self

8. Patients for whom compliance with treatment program may be influenced by financial and third-party payment concerns

■ **Patient education and follow-up goals**

1. Provide support and information

2. **Empower patient to care for self**

3. **Reduce patient's fear, increase his or her self-confidence, improve compliance**

4. **Help patient adjust to treatment**

5. **Increase patient's understanding of treatment goals**

6. **Help patient recognize and control side effects**

7. **Enhance patient's ability to report side effects early**

8. **Document and follow-up to reinforce teaching and to evaluate patient's condition**

■ **Grading of toxicities**

1. *Grading* **is a means of standardization of assessment and documentation of side effects**

2. **To assess toxicity, knowledge of the following is needed**
   ❏ *Which toxicities occurred*
   ❏ *Toxicity severity*
   ❏ *Time of onset*
   ❏ *Duration of effect*
   ❏ *Interventions used to minimize effect*

■ **Systemic toxicities**

1. **Bone marrow suppression**
   ❏ *Most common dose-limiting side effect of chemotherapy*
   ❏ *All hematopoietic cells divide rapidly and are vulnerable to chemotherapy*

❑ *Point of lowest blood count* (nadir) *occurs about 7 to 14 days postchemotherapy*

❑ *Alkylating agents and nitrosoureas are toxic to noncycling and cycling cells*

❑ *Antimetabolites, vinca alkaloids, and antitumor antibiotics are less toxic because they are cycle specific*

❑ *Risk factors for bone marrow suppression*
   ☐ Tumor cells in bone marrow
   ☐ Prior treatment with chemotherapy or radiation
   ☐ Poor nutrition

❑ *Thrombocytopenia*
   ☐ Life span of platelets is 7 to 10 days
   ☐ Thrombocytopenia occurs on days 8 to 14
   ☐ Manifestations of thrombocytopenia
      ▪ Easy bruising
      ▪ Bleeding from gums, nose, or other orifices
      ▪ Petechiae on extremities and pressure points
   ☐ Platelet transfusions are indicated if platelets drop quickly to dangerous level (20,000 /mm^3 or below), or if patient is bleeding

❑ *Anemia*
   ☐ Red blood cells have a life span of 120 days
   ☐ Manifestations of anemia
      ▪ Pallor   ▪ Fatigue
      ▪ Hypotension   ▪ Tachycardia
      ▪ Headache   ▪ Tachypnea
      ▪ Irritability

- ☐ Transfusions are indicated when
    - ▪ Hemoglobin goes below 8 g/100 ml
    - ▪ Patient is symptomatic, e.g., short of breath
    - ▪ Patient is bleeding
- ☐ Consider the growth factor erythropoietin

- ❏ *Neutropenia*
    - ☐ Life span of granulocyte is 6 to 8 hours
    - ☐ Neutropenia usually develops 8 to 12 days after chemotherapy
    - ☐ Chemotherapy is often withheld if white blood cell count (WBC) is below 3000/mm^3 or if absolute neutrophil count (ANC) is below 1500/mm^3
    - ☐ Profound neutropenia (grade 4) is defined as an ANC <500 cells/mm^3
    - ☐ ANC is calculated by multiplying WBC by neutrophil count.

(Segmented neutrophils + bands) × WBC = ANC

    - ☐ Infections from invasion and overgrowth of pathogenic microbes increase in frequency and severity as ANC decreases
    - ☐ Risk of severe infections increases when nadir persists for more than 7 to 10 days
    - ☐ Chemotherapy-induced damage to alimentary canal and respiratory tract mucosa facilitates entry of infecting organisms; 80% of infections arise from endogenous microbial flora
    - ☐ When neutrophil count is less than 500, approximately 20% or more of febrile episodes will have an associated bacteremia caused principally by aerobic gram-negative bacilli and gram-positive cocci

- ☐ Treatment involves culture and broad-spectrum antibiotics for a minimum of 7 days
- ☐ Fever persisting for over 3 days without identification of infected site or organism suggests
  - Nonbacterial cause (may begin antifungal therapy)
  - Resistance to antibiotic
  - Emergence of second bacterial infection
  - Inadequate antibiotic serum and tissue levels
  - Drug fever
  - Infection at avascular site (abscess)
- ☐ Colony-stimulating factors can shorten duration of neutropenia

2. Fatigue

- ❏ *Common and distressing side effect of chemotherapy*

- ❏ *Cause in cancer patient is unknown but may relate to*
  - ☐ Changes in skeletal-muscle protein stores
  - ☐ Metabolite concentration and accumulation
  - ☐ Changes in energy usage or disease pattern
  - ☐ Anemia and psychologic distress
  - ☐ Metabolism of end products of cellular destruction by chemotherapy

- ❏ *Manifestations of fatigue*
  - ☐ Weariness
  - ☐ Weakness
  - ☐ Lack of energy

❏ *Interventions to overcome fatigue*
- ☐ Energy conservation
- ☐ Rest
- ☐ Setting priorities for activities
- ☐ Delegating tasks

3. Gastrointestinal

❏ *Anorexia*

- ☐ Characterized by abnormalities of carbohydrate, protein, and fat metabolism

- ☐ Alterations in food perception, taste, and smell are commonly caused by chemotherapy

- ☐ Anorexia can lead to
  - ■ Decreased calorie intake
  - ■ Weight loss
  - ■ Compromised immune status
  - ■ Decreased macrophage mobilization
  - ■ Depressed lymphocyte function
  - ■ Impaired phagocytosis

- ☐ Management includes
  - ■ Nutritional and physical assessment
  - ■ Dietary diary
  - ■ Consultation with dietitian
  - ■ Dietary plan

- ☐ Degree of anorexia and success of any dietary plan depends on
  - ■ Patient motivation
  - ■ Nutritional status at time of diagnosis
  - ■ Site of cancer
  - ■ Type of treatment
  - ■ Severity of side effects

❏ *Diarrhea*

- ☐ Results from destruction of actively dividing epithelial cells of gastrointestinal (GI) tract

☐ Degree and duration of diarrhea depend on
  ■ Drugs (e.g., 5-fluorouracil, methotrexate)
  ■ Dose
  ■ Nadir
  ■ Frequency of chemotherapy

☐ Abdominal cramps and rectal urgency can evolve into
  ■ Nocturnal diarrhea
  ■ Fecal incontinence
  ■ Lethargy
  ■ Weakness
  ■ Orthostatic hypotension
  ■ Fluid and electrolyte imbalance

☐ Prolonged diarrhea will cause
  ■ Dehydration
  ■ Nutritional malabsorption
  ■ Circulatory collapse

☐ Management often includes
  ■ Temporarily discontinuing chemotherapy
  ■ Low-residue, high-caloric, high-protein diet
  ■ Pharmacologic measures
  ■ Stool cultures to rule out infectious process
  ■ *Clostridium difficile* has been reported in patients receiving chemotherapy who have had prior antibiotic exposure
  ■ Antidiarrheal agents are not given to counteract diarrhea resulting from infection, since these agents slow passage of stool through intestines, prolonging mucosa's exposure to organism's toxins

- Pharmacologic intervention for diarrhea includes

  Anticholinergic drugs to reduce gastric secretions and decrease intestinal peristalsis

  Opiate therapy binds to receptors on smooth muscle of bowel, slowing down intestinal motility and increasing fluid absorption

  Octreotide acetate
     Synthetic analog of hormone octapeptide

     Inhibits release of gut hormones including serotonin and gastrin from GI tract

     Prolongs intestinal transit time, increasing intestinal water and electrolyte transport, and decreasing GI bloodflow

- ❏ *Constipation*
  - ☐ Infrequent, excessively hard and dry bowel movements result from decrease in rectal filling or emptying
  - ☐ Risk factors
    - Narcotic analgesics
    - Decrease in physical activity
    - Low-fiber diet
    - Decrease in fluid intake
    - Poor dentition in elderly population
    - Bed rest

- Diminished rectal emptying due to vincristine or vinblastine therapy; these drugs cause autonomic nerve dysfunction and symptoms may include peripheral nerve dysfunction

☐ Prevention of constipation

- Prophylactic stool softener prior to beginning vincristine or vinblastine therapy
- Increase fiber, fluids, and physical activity
- Notify physician if more than 3 days has passed without bowel movement since impaction, ileus, or obstipation can occur

❏ *Nausea and vomiting*

☐ Vomiting center (VC) contains neurotransmitter receptors sensitive to chemical toxins in blood and cerebrospinal fluid

☐ Major receptors are

- Dopamine
- Serotonin (5-HT3) in central nervous system (CNS) and GI tract
- Muscarinic cholinergic in chemoreceptor trigger zone
- Muscarinic in VC vestibular apparatus
- Efferent vagal motor nuclei
- Histamine in VC and vestibular apparatus

☐ Emesis can be induced by

- Stimulation of VC
- Obstruction, irritation, inflammation, or delayed gastric emptying
- Conditioned anticipatory responses

- ☐ Nausea
    - Subjective conscious recognition of urge to vomit
    - Manifested by unpleasant wavelike sensation in epigastric area, at back of throat, or throughout abdomen
    - Mediated by autonomic nervous system and accompanied by symptoms such as tachycardia, perspiration, lightheadedness, dizziness, pallor, excess salivation, and weakness
- ☐ Retching
    - Rhythmic and spasmodic movement involving diaphragm and abdominal muscles
    - Controlled by respiratory center in brainstem near VC
    - Negative intrathoracic pressure and positive abdominal pressure result in unproductive retching
    - When negative pressure becomes positive, vomiting occurs
- ☐ Vomiting
    - Somatic process performed by respiratory muscles causing forceful oral expulsion of gastric, duodenal, or jejunal contents
- ☐ Classifications of nausea and vomiting
    - *Acute:* Nausea and vomiting 1 to 2 hours after treatment
    - *Delayed:* Nausea and vomiting persist or develop 24 hours after chemotherapy
    - Delayed nausea and vomiting are less common if acute emesis is prevented

- ■ *Anticipatory:* Nausea and vomiting occur as result of classic operant conditioning from stimuli associated with chemotherapy
- ■ Conditioned responses experienced after few sessions of chemotherapy
- ■ Occur most commonly when efforts to control emesis are unsuccessful
- □ Prevention and management
  - ■ Identification of risk factors for nausea and vomiting are important strategies
  - ■ Risk factors include

    Emetic potential of drug(s)

    Onset and duration of emetic response

    Dose of drug

    Schedule of drug

    Age: Younger are more susceptible

    Prior chemotherapy

    Anxiety

    Gender: Women more than men
  - ■ Management strategies

    Treat prophylactically, prior to chemotherapeutic treatment

    Combination antiemetic therapy

    Employ behavior strategies; e.g., progressive muscle relaxation, hypnosis, and systematic desensitization

■ Organ toxicities

1. Cardiotoxicity

- ❏ *Acute cardiac toxicity*
  - □ Characterized by transient electrocardiogram changes

- ❑ Occurs in about 10% of patients receiving chemotherapy

❑ *Chronic cardiac toxicity*
- ❑ Characterized by onset of symptoms occurring weeks or months after therapy
- ❑ Cardiomyopathy is irreversible
- ❑ Congestive heart failure presents as low-voltage QRS complex
- ❑ Less than 5% of patients develop chronic cardiotoxicity

❑ *Signs and symptoms*
- ❑ Nonproductive cough
- ❑ Dyspnea
- ❑ Pedal edema

❑ *Risk factors*
- ❑ Anthracyclines directly damage myocyte of heart
- ❑ Total cumulative dose of doxorubicin is 550 mg/m^2 and 600 mg/m^2 for daunorubicin
- ❑ If mediastinal radiation has been given, dose is reduced to 450 mg/m^2
- ❑ High doses of cyclophosphamide or 5-fluorouracil increase risk for cardiac damage

❑ *Prevention*
- ❑ Limit total dose of anthracycline
- ❑ Low-dose continuous infusions minimize cardiac toxicity
- ❑ Administer chemoprotectants if appropriate
- ❑ Utilize less cardiotoxic analogs if possible

- ❏ *Management*
  - ☐ Monitor ECG and radionuclide scan to evaluate heart function
  - ☐ Instruct patient to conserve energy
  - ☐ Manage fluid retention and minimize sodium intake
  - ☐ Digitalis therapy may enhance cardiac output
  - ☐ Diuretics may be useful to decrease cardiac load
  - ☐ Oxygen may be useful to manage dyspnea

2. Neurotoxicity

- ❏ *Chemotherapy-induced neurotoxicity may result in direct or indirect damage to CNS, peripheral nervous system, cranial nerves, or any combination of the three*
- ❏ *CNS damage primarily involves cerebellum; this damage produces altered reflexes, unsteady gait, ataxia, and confusion*
- ❏ *Damage to peripheral nervous system produces paralysis or loss of movement and sensation to those areas affected by the particular nerve*
- ❏ *Damage to autonomic nervous system causes ileus, impotence, or urinary retention*
- ❏ *Drugs most commonly associated with neurotoxicity*
  - ☐ Vincristine
    - ■ Peripheral neuropathy
    - ■ Myalgias, loss of deep tendon reflexes at ankle, progressing to complete areflexia

- Distal symmetric sensory loss, motor weakness, footdrop, and muscle atrophy

- Autonomic neuropathy can also occur with vincristine and is characterized by ileus, constipation, impotence, urinary retention, or postural hypotension

☐ Cisplatin

- Damages large-diameter fibers of neural tissues, causing sensory changes

- Paresthesias of hands and feet are common

- Sensory ataxia

- High-tone hearing loss

☐ Taxol

- Peripheral neuropathy

- Myalgias and arthralgias are dose-dependent

- Autonomic neuropathy

- Symptoms gradually improve after cessation of therapy

☐ Other drugs associated with neurotoxicity

- Ifosfamide
- High-dose methotrexate
- High-dose cytarabine
- 5-fluorouracil

☐ Prevention

- Neurologic assessment prior to treatment

- Sedatives, tranquilizers, and antiemetics might increase toxicity

- Dose modification may be necessary to prevent irreversible damage

3. Pulmonary toxicity

❑ *Chemotherapy can damage endothelial cells, resulting in pneumonitis*

❑ *Long-term exposure to chemotherapy causes extensive alteration of pulmonary parenchyma*

❑ *Presenting symptoms*
- ☐ Dyspnea
- ☐ Unproductive cough
- ☐ Bilateral basilar rales
- ☐ Tachypnea

❑ *Risk factors*
- ☐ Age: Very young and elderly
- ☐ Preexisting lung disease
- ☐ History of smoking
- ☐ Cumulative dose
- ☐ Long-term therapy
- ☐ Mediastinal radiation
- ☐ High inspired concentration of oxygen

❑ *Drugs commonly associated with pulmonary toxicity*
- ☐ Bleomycin: Cumulative dose should not exceed 400 to 450 units; it induces interstitial changes with hyperplasia
- ☐ Cytarabine directly damages pneumocytes
- ☐ Mitomycin C causes diffuse alveolar damage
- ☐ Cyclophosphamide causes endothelial swelling

❑ *Prevention and management*
- ☐ Symptoms of pulmonary toxicity
  - ▪ Low-grade fever
  - ▪ Nonproductive cough
  - ▪ Dyspnea
  - ▪ Tachycardia

- Diffuse basilar crackles
- Wheezing
- Pleural rub
- Fatigue

□ Management
- Conservation of energy
- Steroids
- Diuretics

4. Hepatotoxicity

❑ *Chemotherapy can cause damage to parenchymal cells*

❑ *Obstruction to hepatic bloodflow results in fatty changes, hepatocellular necrosis, and veno-occlusive disease*

❑ *Risk factors for veno-occlusive disease*
   □ Increased age
   □ Hepatitis
   □ Elevated serum glutamic oxaloacetic transaminase (SGOT)

❑ *Clinical signs of veno-occlusive disease*
   □ Weight gain
   □ Jaundice
   □ Abdominal pain
   □ Hepatomegaly
   □ Encephalopathy
   □ Elevated bilirubin and SGOT values

❑ *Chemotherapy drugs commonly associated with liver toxicity*
   □ Methotrexate   □ Nitrosoureas
   □ 6-Mercaptopurine   □ Etoposide
   □ Cytarabine

❑ *Symptoms of hepatotoxicity*
  ☐ Elevated liver function tests
  ☐ Chemical hepatitis
  ☐ Jaundice
  ☐ Ascites
  ☐ Decreased albumin
  ☐ Cirrhosis

5. Hemorrhagic cystitis

❑ *Results from damage to bladder mucosa caused by acrolein, a metabolite of cyclophosphamide and ifosfamide*

❑ *Symptoms of hemorrhagic cystitis*
  ☐ Microscopic hematuria
  ☐ Transient irritative urination
  ☐ Dysuria
  ☐ Suprapubic pain
  ☐ Hemorrhage

❑ *Risk factors*
  ☐ High doses of ifosfamide or cyclophosphamide

❑ *Prevention and management*
  ☐ Adequate hydration
  ☐ Empty bladder frequently
  ☐ Mesna therapy
  ☐ Test urine for occult blood (Hemastik)

6. Nephrotoxicity

❑ *Damage to kidneys is caused either by direct renal cell damage or obstructive nephropathy; i.e., tumor lysis syndrome or uric acid nephropathy*

❑ *Risk factors*
  ☐ Elderly patient

- ☐ Preexisting renal disease
- ☐ Poor nutritional status
- ☐ Dehydration
- ☐ Large tumor mass
- ☐ High cumulative dose of nephrotoxic drug
- ☐ Concomitant administration of aminoglycoside therapy

❏ *Symptoms*
- ☐ Increased blood urea nitrogen and creatinine
- ☐ Oliguria
- ☐ Azotemia
- ☐ Proteinuria
- ☐ Hyperuricemia
- ☐ Hypomagnesemia
- ☐ Hypocalcemia

❏ *Drugs commonly associated with nephrotoxicity*
- ☐ *Cisplatin:* Damages renal cell
- ☐ *Methotrexate:* Damage occurs because drug precipitates out in an acid environment to obstruct renal tubules
- ☐ *Streptozocin:* Directly damages tubules, causing tubular atrophy
- ☐ *Nitrosoureas:* Cause delayed renal failure: azotemia and proteinuria followed by progressive renal failure
- ☐ *Mitomycin C:* Renal failure and microangiopathic hemolytic anemia occur in approximately 20% of patients who have received cumulative dose of 100 mg or more

❏ *Prevention of nephrotoxicity*
  ☐ Evaluate renal status prior to therapy
  ☐ Adequately hydrate patient
  ☐ Encourage patient to drink 3,000 cc of fluid per day
  ☐ Decrease uric acid production with allopurinol in patients with high tumor load
  ☐ Ensure that patient receiving methotrexate has pretreatment with sodium bicarbonate to alkalinize urine

7. Gonadal toxicity

❏ *Chemotherapy causes gonadal changes*
  ☐ Gonadal failure
  ☐ Infertility
  ☐ Premature menopause

❏ *Risk factors for gonadal toxicity*
  ☐ Age: Women over 30 are less likely to regain ovarian function because they have fewer oocytes with aging
  ☐ Cycle nonspecific agents are most toxic and include

  - Busulfan
  - Nitrogen mustard
  - Chlorambucil
  - Melphalan
  - Procarbazine

  ☐ Drug-induced testicular damage results in azospermia, oligospermia, and abnormalities of semen volume, motility
  ☐ Sperm banking is an option for men to preserve their ability to produce children

8. Secondary and therapy-related cancers

❏ *Risk factors*

☐ Long-term survivors are at highest risk for second primary cancer

☐ Alkylating agents are most often implicated as risk factors for second malignancies

☐ Long-term survivors and their children should be monitored for their lifetimes

Suggested Readings

1. Camp-Sorrell D: Chemotherapy: Toxicity management. In Groenwald SL, Frogge MH, Goodman M, Yarbro CH, (eds.): *Cancer Nursing: Principles and Practice* (3rd ed.). Boston: Jones and Bartlett, 1993, pp. 331–365.

2. Nail LM, Jones LS, Greene D, et al: Use and perceived efficacy of self-care activities in patients receiving chemotherapy. *Oncol Nurs Forum* 18:883–887, 1991.

3. Maxwell MB, Maher KE: Chemotherapy-induced myelosuppression. *Semin Oncol Nurs* 8:113–123, 1992.

4. Hoagland HC: Hematologic complications of cancer chemotherapy. In Perry MC (ed.): *The Chemotherapy Source Book.* Baltimore: Williams & Wilkins, 1992, pp. 498–507.

5. Knobf MK, Durivage HJ: Chemotherapy: Principles of practice. In Groenwald SL, Frogge MH, Goodman M, and Yarbro CH (eds.): *Cancer Nursing: Principles and Practice* (3rd ed.). Boston: Jones and Bartlett, 1993, pp. 271–292.

6. Krakoff IH: Cancer chemotherapeutic and biologic agents. *CA J* 41:264–278, 1991.

7. Reymann RE: Chemotherapy: Principles of administration. In Groenwald SL, Frogge MH, Goodman M, Yarbro CH (eds.): *Cancer Nursing: Principles and Practice* (3rd ed.). Boston: Jones and Bartlett, 1993, 293–330.

8. Yarbro CH: Nursing implications in the administration of cancer chemotherapy. In Perry MC (ed.): *The Chemotherapy Source Book.* Baltimore: Williams & Wilkins, 1992, pp. 873–883.

9. Goodman M: Delivery of cancer chemotherapy. In Baird S, McCorkle R, Grant M (eds.): *Cancer Nursing: A Comprehensive Textbook.* Philadelphia: Saunders, 1991, p. 311.

10. Wickham R, Purl S, Welker D: Long-term central venous catheters: Issues for care. *Semin Oncol Nurs* 8:133–147, 1991.

■11■
Biotherapy

Overview

- ■ Biotherapy is based on hypothesis that immune system can be manipulated to restore, augment, or modulate its function
- ■ Evidence from animal and human trials indicates that under proper circumstances, malignant tumors are susceptible to immunologic rejection
- ■ Biologic response modifiers (BRMs) are soluble substances capable of altering immune system with either stimulatory or suppressive effect
- ■ Three major categories of BRMs
1. Agents that restore, augment, or modulate host's immunologic mechanisms
2. Agents that have direct antitumor activity

3. Agents that have other biologic effects (agents interfering with tumor cells' ability to survive or metastasize; differentiating agents or agents affecting cell transformation

Types of Immunotherapy and Their Side Effects

■ **Antibody therapy (serotherapy)**

1. Promotes specific targeting of cells through antibody-antigen response

2. Monoclonal antibodies (MAbs) may be used alone or in combination with radioisotopes, toxins, or chemotherapeutic drugs (immunoconjugates) to stain, destroy, or identify cells with specific antigens on their cell surfaces

3. Also used in vitro to remove tumor cells from bone marrow before autologous bone marrow transplantation and in conjunction with other BRMs

4. Toxicities most often occur within 2 to 8 hours following antibody administration and include

   ❏ *Anaphylaxis (infrequent)*
   □ Signs and symptoms
     ■ Predicted by presence of generalized flush or urticaria followed by pallor or cyanosis, or both

- Patient may complain of tickle in throat or impending doom
- Complaints of bronchospasm are common
- Hypotension and unconsciousness may result

☐ Nursing measures

- Stop antibody infusion immediately
- Assess patient's vital signs frequently
- Alert physician
- Administer 0.3 cc aqueous 1:1000 epinephrine subcutaneously if patient is conscious and has detectable blood pressure
- For patients who cannot be aroused, epinephrine 1:10,000 is administered by intravenous push
- Additional therapeutic measures may include

    Administration of oxygen

    Administration of antihistamines, corticosteroids, and aminophylline

    Cardiopulmonary resuscitation

❏ *Fever*	❏ *Urticaria*
❏ *Chills*	❏ *Pruritus*
❏ *Diaphoresis*	❏ *Dyspnea*
❏ *Rigors*	❏ *Nausea*
❏ *Malaise*	❏ *Vomiting*
❏ *Pallor*	❏ *Diarrhea*
❏ *Weakness*	❏ *Hypotension*
❏ *Generalized erythema*	

■ Cytokines

1. **Substances released from activated immune system cells that affect behavior of other cells**

2. **Activate variety of biologic activities that may alter growth and metastasis of cancer cells**

3. **May be administered directly to patients for control of cancer, or may be used to manipulate immune response in vitro to generate products used to treat individuals with cancer**

4. **Examples include**

   ❏ *Interferon (IFN)*
   - □ Naturally occurring cytokines that interfere with virus activity in cells
   - □ Have antiproliferative effect
   - □ Three major types
     - ▪ α-IFN
     - ▪ β-IFN
     - ▪ γ-IFN
   - □ Each type originates from different cell and has distinct biologic and chemical properties
   - □ Routes of administration
     - ▪ Subcutaneous
     - ▪ Intramuscular
     - ▪ Intravenous bolus
     - ▪ Intravenous continuous infusion
     - ▪ Intrathecal
     - ▪ Intralesional
     - ▪ Intracavity
   - □ Route significantly alters pharmacokinetics
   - □ Toxicities are dose-related and include

- Flulike syndrome: Fever, chills, malaise, fatigue

- Central nervous system (CNS): Headache, lethargy, somnolence, seizures, confusion, impaired concentration

- Renal/hepatic: Elevated transaminase, proteinuria

- Reproductive: Impotence, decreased libido

- Gastrointestinal (GI): Nausea, vomiting, diarrhea, anorexia/weight loss

- Hematologic: Leukopenia, thrombocytopenia, anemia

- Cardiovascular: Hypotension, tachycardia, arrhythmias, myocardial ischemia

- Integumentary: Alopecia, irritation at injection site

☐ Treatment is symptomatic

❏ *Interleukins (IL)*

☐ Regulatory substances produced by lymphocytes and monocytes

☐ Variety of immunoregulative biologic activities that stimulate proliferation and maturation of immune cells

☐ Types include

- Interleukin-1

    Potential clinical applications

    Prevention or reversal of iatrogenic neutropenia

    Reversal of thrombocytopenia

    Bone marrow transplantation

    Antiproliferative effects

    Infectious disease

Dysmyelopoietic states

Combination therapy with other cytokines

Administered subcutaneously to rotating sites on arms, abdomen, and thighs, with ice applied after injection to prevent bleeding

Toxicities include

Fever	Asthenia
Chills	Anorexia
Headache	Hypotension
Nausea and vomiting	Myalgia
Tachycardia	Diarrhea

Hypotension is dose-limiting toxicity

- Interleukin-2

  Supports proliferation and augmentation of natural killer cells

  Is critical for generation of lymphokine-activated killer (LAK) cells

  Augments various other T-cell functions

  Activates cytotoxic effector cells that produce cytokines

  Used in conjunction with LAK cells or tumor-infiltrating lymphocytes, in combination with other biologic agents, and in combination with chemotherapeutic agents

  Produces objective tumor responses in 15% to 45% of patients with renal cell carcinoma and malignant melanoma

Toxicities are multisystem and may be life-threatening; however, all are usually reversible within 24 to 96 hours after therapy

CNS

Disorientation

Monitor for overt and subtle changes in mental status

IL-2 held or discontinued if agitation, restlessness, or increased anxiety are present

Some patients progress rapidly to somnolence, disorientation, or severe agitation, and require restraints

Symptoms resolve within 24 to 48 hours after therapy ceases

Cardiovascular/pulmonary

Marked cardiovascular and pulmonary toxicities occur when IL-2 is administered at high dose

Capillary leak syndrome, characterized by marked extravascular fluid shifts, consistently occurs

Peripheral vasodilation occurs, with significant decrease in systemic vascular resistance and increase in heart rate

Hypotension begins soon after onset of treatment

Plasma protein fraction or albumin is administered

Dopamine HCl or phenylephrine HCl (Neosynephrine) is administered to keep systolic blood pressure greater than 90

Tachycardia occurs as compensatory response

Cardiac dysrhythmias occur in 10% of patients

Respond to traditional medical management with digoxin or verapamil

Daily EKGs and increased vital sign monitoring for patients taking vasopressors are indicated

Transient cardiac ischemia has been reported; myocardial infarction is rare, but has been reported

Pulmonary congestion is common

Patients may require oxygen therapy

Oxygen saturation is monitored by pulse oximetry

Patients with histories of cardiac or pulmonary dysfunction are not eligible for treatment with IL-2

Renal

Oliguria, anuria, azotemia, and elevations of serum creatinine and blood urea nitrogen levels occur

Progressive respiratory alkalosis and hypophosphatemia, hypocalcemia, and hypomagnesemia may occur

Low-dose dopamine assists with renal perfusion

Normal renal function returns spontaneously after IL-2 therapy is stopped

Patients with prior nephrectomy are at high risk and should be monitored closely

GI

Nausea and vomiting are controlled with antiemetics

Diarrhea is common and may require administration of bicarbonate

Stomatitis is frequent but not severe

Malaise and anorexia are not treatment-limiting

Hepatic

Increased levels of serum bilirubin and liver enzymes, and progressive hypoalbuminemia occur with IL-2 therapy

Mild to moderate hepatomegaly without abdominal tenderness occurs commonly

Hematologic

Severe anemia occurs in 77% of patients who receive IL-2

Warrants transfusion of packed red blood cells

Thrombocytopenia is common, but platelet therapy is rarely indicated

No severe coagulopathies have been reported

Integumentary

Diffuse erythematous pruritic rash progresses to desquamation in IL-2

Desquamation can be severe, involving soles of feet, palms of hands, and moist, intertriginous areas

Flulike syndrome

Patients develop fever, chills, rigors, and malaise

Managed by prophylactic administration of acetaminophen, diphenhydramine, and indomethacin

If fever or chills develop, meperidine 25 to 50 mg intravenous push or lorazepam 1 to 2 mg intravenous push is effective

Endocrinologic

Twenty percent of patients receiving high doses of IL-2/LAK develop hypothyroidism

Other IL-2 endocrinologic effects include increases in blood levels of adrenocorticotropic hormone, cortisol, prolactin, growth hormone, and acute-phase reactant C-reactive protein

LAK cell reaction

Mild to severe chills followed by transient fever have been reported within 0.5–1 hour after first administration; reactions are less severe with subsequent administration

- Tumor necrosis factor

Produced by macrophages

Cytotoxic or cytostatic on tumor cells with no effect on normal cells

Therapeutic effects under clinical investigation

Administered

By intravenous bolus

By continuous intravenous infusion

Sub cutaneously

By intramuscular injection

Optimal route has not been established

Clinical toxicities are similar to IL-2

- Colony-stimulating factors (CSF)

Regulate hematopoiesis

In culture, stimulate growth of colonies of maturing blood cells from their hematopoietic precursors

Used prophylactically or therapeutically in treatment of disease states in which myelosuppression, anemia, and thrombocytopenia limit therapeutic treatment options

Allow increased or scheduled doses of chemotherapeutic agents to be given with long-term myelosuppression

Effective in other hematologic diseases such as acquired immunodeficiency syndrome, in which abnormalities of blood cell components exist

CSFs include erythropoietin, granulocyte-CSF (G-CSF), granulocyte-macrophage-CSF (GM-CSF), IL-3, and macrophage-CSF

Examples include

Erythropoietin

Treats anemia related to cancer

Administered subcutaneously

Response seen (increased hematocrit) within 14 to 21 days following initiation of treatment

Minimal side effects

G-CSF

Used to treat chemotherapy-induced neutropenia

Administered subcutaneously, or short intravenous infusion

Side effects include flulike syndrome with fever, myalgias and headache, generalized rash, and bone pain

GM-CSF

Broader spectrum than G-CSF

Stimulates both macrophages and neutropenia

Decreases requirement for platelet and red cell transfusions in addition to its effect on granulocytes

Permits dose intensification and enhances myeloprotection before and after chemotherapy

Food and Drug Administration–approved for treatment of neutropenia associated with autologous bone marrow transplantation

Administered by subcutaneous or intravenous infusion

Side effects include

Flulike syndrome (fever, chills, rigors, myalgias, headache, fatigue)

Facial flushing

Generalized rash

Inflammation at injection site

Leukocytosis

Eosinophilia

Dyspnea

Bone pain

Fluid retention

Nursing Management

■ **BRM administration requires signed statement of informed consent for all research protocols**

1. **Nurse is involved in discussion with patient and family**

■ Nurses must be familiar with agents used and their common toxicities to predict occurrence and severity of toxicities

■ Nurses provide education to patient about treatment and expected toxicities

■ Nurses provide psychosocial support during treatment

Suggested Readings

1. Jassak PF: Biotherapy. In Groenwald SL, Frogge, MH, Goodman M, Yarbro CH (eds.): *Cancer Nursing: Principles and Practice* (3rd ed.). Boston: Jones and Bartlett, 1993, pp. 366–392.

2. Rosenberg SA: The immunotherapy and gene therapy of cancer. *J Clin Oncol* 10:180–199, 1992.

3. Carter P, Engleking C, Rumsey K, et al: *Biological Response Modifier Guidelines. Recommendations for Nursing Education and Practice.* Pittsburgh: Oncology Nursing Society, 1989.

▪ 12 ▪
Bone Marrow Transplantation

Overview

■ Types of Bone Marrow Transplantation (BMT)

1. Syngeneic

❑ *Donor is an identical twin (perfect human leukocyte antigen [HLA] match)*

2. Allogeneic

❑ *Depends on availability of HLA-matched donor*

❑ *Graft-versus-host disease (GVHD) is unique complication*

❑ *Diseases treated with allogeneic BMT include*
   ☐ Acute and chronic leukemias
   ☐ Lymphomas
   ☐ Myeloma
   ☐ Aplastic anemia
   ☐ Immunologic deficiencies
   ☐ Inborn errors of metabolism

❑ *Most appropriate donor depends on tissue typing of HLA*

❑ *Donor marrow is harvested in operating room*

3. Autologous bone marrow transplant (ABMT)

❑ *Patient receives his or her own marrow*

❑ *Diseases treated with ABMT include*
  - ☐ Acute and chronic leukemias
  - ☐ Lymphomas
  - ☐ Some solid tumors

❑ *Advantages*
  - ☐ Absence of GVHD
  - ☐ Fewer BMT-related toxicities

❑ *Harvested marrow is purged to remove malignant cells before reinfusion*

4. Autologous: Peripheral Stem Cell Transplant (PSCT)

❑ *Candidates are patients ineligible for ABMT because their marrow is hypoplastic or metastatic*

❑ *Peripheral stem cells are collected by apheresis*

❑ *Cells are cryopreserved for infusion at later date*

BMT Process

■ **Candidates and donor require comprehensive evaluations**

■ **Pretransplant conditioning regimens involve high-dose chemotherapy alone or with total-body irradiation**

■ **Marrow is infused through central lumen catheter over several hours**

■ **Toxicities and complications most severe until marrow graft becomes functional**

Acute Complications of BMT

■ **Gastrointestinal (GI) toxicity**

1. **Occurs 0 to 28 days after BMT**

2. **Clinical manifestations include**
   ❏ *Mucositis*
   ❏ *Nausea and vomiting*
   ❏ *Diarrhea*

■ **Acute GVHD**

1. **Occurs 10 to 70 days after allogeneic BMT**

2. **Clinical manifestations**
   ❏ *Maculopapular rash progressing to erythroderma with desquamation*

   ❏ *Elevated liver enzymes, right upper-quadrant pain, hepatomegaly, and jaundice*

   ❏ *Green, watery diarrhea and abdominal cramping*

   ❏ *Anorexia, nausea, vomiting*

3. **Prophylaxis and approaches to care**
   ❏ *Administer cyclosporine and methotrexate to inhibit T-lymphocytes*

❑ *Administer antithymocyte globulin*

❑ *Assess patient's integumentary system*

❑ *Monitor liver function tests, guaiac stool test, patient's weight, intake and output, and electrolytes*

❑ *Assess patient's nutritional status*

▨ Hematologic complications

1. Bleeding can occur from all body orifices

❑ *Requires irradiated blood products, HLA-matched platelets*

❑ *Follow appropriate nursing interventions for bleeding*

2. Hemorrhagic cystitis from high-dose cyclophosphamide

❑ *Assess patient's fluid intake and force fluids*

▨ Renal insufficiency

1. Occurs 1 to 50 days after BMT

2. Early clinical manifestations include

❑ *Anuria*
❑ *Acid-base imbalances*
❑ *Doubling of baseline creatinine*

▨ Veno-occlusive disease of liver

1. Almost exclusive to BMT

2. Occurs 6 to 15 days after BMT

3. Clinical manifestations

❑ *Fluid retention*

❑ *Sudden weight gain*

❑ *Abdominal distention*

❑ *Right upper-quadrant pain*

❑ *Increased bilirubin and serum glutamic oxaloacetic transaminase (SGOT)*

❑ *Hepatomegaly*

❑ *Encephalopathy*

4. **No known treatment; provide symptom management and supportive care**

■ **Infection**

1. **Most common sites of infections are**
   ❑ *GI tract*
   ❑ *Oropharynx*
   ❑ *Lung*
   ❑ *Skin*
   ❑ *Indwelling catheter sites*

2. **Most common infections from days 0 to 30 are**
   ❑ *Bacterial: gram-negative and gram-positive*
   ❑ *Herpes simplex I and II*
   ❑ *Candida and Aspergillus*

3. **Most common infections from days 30 to 90 are**
   ❑ *Cytomegalovirus (CMV)*
      ☐ CMV pneumonia a common occurrence

   ❑ *Gram-positive bacteria*

   ❑ *Pneumocystis carinii*

4. **Most common infections after engraftment are**
   - ❏ *Encapsulated bacteria*
   - ❏ *Varicella zoster*

Clinical Management of BMT Outpatient

■ Hospital discharge after BMT averages 30 to 35 days but may be shorter with ABMT and PSCT.

■ Common discharge criteria are

1. Availability of 24-hour outpatient medical care

2. Oral intake 25 to 50% of baseline nutrient requirements

3. No more than 2500 ml of parenteral fluid required every 24 hours

4. Nausea and vomiting controlled

5. Diarrhea controlled at <500 ml/day

6. Platelet count supportable at 5000 to 15,000/mm^3

7. Granulocytes >500/mm^3 for 24 hours

8. Hematocrit >25%

9. Patient tolerating medications by mouth

10. Family support at home

■ **Patients experience at least 3 months of severe immunodeficiency**

■ **Immune function generally returns in 6 to 9 months**

■ **Immune recovery delayed in allogeneic patients with chronic GVHD**

■ **Numerous tests and evaluations are needed for follow-up**

Late Complications of BMT

■ **Chronic GVHD**

1. **Major cause of morbidity after allogeneic BMT**

2. **Onset is 100 to 400 days after BMT**

3. **Clinical manifestations**

❏ *Skin involvement*
   □ Itching, burning rash
   □ Erythema
   □ Hypopigmentation and hyperpigmentation
   □ Fibrosis

❏ *Liver disorders*
   □ Jaundice
   □ Abnormal liver function tests

❏ *Oral involvement*
- □ Pain, burning, dryness
- □ Loss of taste
- □ Stomatitis
- □ Dental decay
- □ Xerostomia

❏ *Ocular involvement*
- □ Burning and itching
- □ Dry eyes

❏ *GI tract*
- □ Anorexia, weight loss
- □ Dysphagia

❏ *Vaginal involvement*
- □ Inflammation
- □ Dryness
- □ Stricture formation

4. Treatment

❏ *Long-term administration of cyclosporine with or without prednisone*

❏ *Symptom-related supportive measures*

▪ Late complications of high-dose chemotherapy or total-body irradiation are

1. **Gonadal dysfunction**

2. **Thyroid dysfunction**

3. **Cataracts**

4. **Dental decay**

5. **Radiation nephritis**

6. **Impaired memory and learning disorders**

7. **Second malignancy**

Psychosocial Issues

- Stresses encountered with each phase of BMT process

- Counselling and education promote realistic expectations

- Support should be available for nurses

- Moral and ethical issues include

1. Allocation of resources
2. Competitive selection of marrow recipients
3. Life support in irreversible organ failure

- Research studies on quality of life after BMT are emerging

Suggested Readings

1. Buchsel PC: Bone marrow transplantation. In Groenwald SL, Frogge MH, Goodman M, Yarbro CH (eds.): *Cancer Nursing: Principles and Practice.* Boston: Jones and Bartlett, 1993, pp. 393–434.

2. Buchsel PC: Ambulatory care for the bone marrow transplant patient. In Buchsel PC, Yarbro CH (eds.): *Oncology Nursing in the Ambulatory Setting.* Boston: Jones and Bartlett, 1993, pp. 185–216.

3. Franco T, Gould DA: Allogeneic bone marrow transplantation. *Semin Oncol Nurs* 10: 3–11, 1994.

4. Whedon MB (ed.): *Bone Marrow Transplantation: Principles, Practice, and Nursing Insights.* Boston: Jones and Bartlett, 1991.

PART III

Psychological and Social Dimensions of Cancer

■ 13 ■
Psychosocial Aspects of Cancer

Characteristics of Cancer

■ Psychosocial responses to cancer experience are determined by

1. Characteristics of cancer

2. Person with or at risk for cancer

3. Social system and environment of significance to individual

■ Cancer poses a universal threat

1. Cancer is among the most feared of all diseases because

   ❏ *It occurs without warning*

   ❏ *It spreads without control*

   ❏ *It is incurable beyond a certain point*

   ❏ *It is associated with pain and discomfort*

❏ *It generates social and professional attitudes of hopelessness*

❏ *It is difficult to diagnose*

❏ *It sometimes requires mutilative surgery*

❏ *It has an unknown cause*

❏ *Cooperation with treatment does not necessarily lead to successful outcomes*

2. **Perceived absence of pathology is never certain; there is constant threat of cancer that can alter achievement of societal roles and self-actualization**

■ **The stigma of cancer persists**

1. **Individuals with cancer experience**

❏ *Insurance cancellation*

❏ *Job discrimination*

❏ *Problems with reintegration into school and workplace*

■ **Disease and treatment are marked by uncertainty**

1. **Uncertainty is compounded by**

❏ *Delays in diagnosis*
❏ *Unpredictable prognoses*
❏ *Early death*

■ Cancer trajectory is manifest by chronicity

1. Simple crisis resolution models are not sufficient to address scope of problems encountered

2. People with cancer are confronted with continuing series of stressors, rather than a single, time-limited crisis

3. Lifelong fear of recurrence is one of the most disruptive aspects

4. Outcome goal is to maintain quality of life throughout all phases of illness

5. "Recovery model" of chronic disease of cancer focuses on survival versus dying and emphasizes self-care over professional intervention

6. Self-care and social and professional support strengthen recovery and influence quality of life throughout recovery process

Individual Responses to Cancer

■ Help-seeking responses

1. Patients search for psychosocial resources to deal with actual or potential threat of cancer

2. Patients do self-appraisal and then expand spheres to significant others and finally to members of health care professions

3. Return to health is manifest by professional's returning responsibility for health care to family and ultimately to patient

■ Culturally determined responses

1. Specific culture of individual shapes his or her view of health

2. Health and illness responses and behaviors are acquired through lifelong socialization

3. Cancer can challenge lifelong values and beliefs and may result in changed cognitive, affective, and behavioral responses

■ Stress, emotions, and coping responses

1. Stress is

❑ *Relationship between person and environment in which demands tax or exceed person's resources*

❑ *System of interdependent processes including appraisal and coping, that mediate frequency, intensity, duration, and type of psychologic and somatic responses*

❑ *Not an inherent characteristic of person or environment*

2. Coping

❑ *Consists of cognitive and behavioral efforts to manage stress*

❏ *Responses used initially by patients may be outmoded as disease and its treatment progress*
  □ Past experience with stressful situations affects one's ability to adapt to current stress
  □ Unresolved past stresses may make current stressors difficult or impossible to cope with

■ Anxiety

1. **Described, with depression, as most common psychosocial reaction experienced by people with cancer**

2. **Defined as**

   ❏ *Individual perceives certain beliefs, values, and conditions essential to secure existence*

   ❏ *Individual experiences nonspecific internal or external stimuli perceived as threats to secure existence*

   ❏ *Individual responds to perceived threat affectively with increased level of arousal associated with vague, unpleasant, and uneasy feelings defined as anxiety*

3. **Individuals with cancer have higher levels of anxiety than individuals with nonmalignant condition**

4. **Anxiety increases at diagnosis and remains elevated in varying levels throughout course of treatment**

5. **Anxiety at minimal or moderate levels may be motivating for patient**

6. Interventions

❏ *Help patient to recognize various manifestations*

❏ *Determine if patient desires to do anything about response*

❏ *Activate coping strategies to control anxiety levels*
  ☐ Teach patient through formal and informal educational programs
  ☐ Assist in problem solving through counselling
  ☐ Role model with anxiety-reducing techniques such as relaxation training or music therapy

❏ *Refer patient to support groups within care institution and community*

■ Depression

1. When depressed, the

❏ *Individual perceives certain goals for future and attributes possibilities for success to self*

❏ *Individual's attempts to attain goals are blocked*

❏ *Individual attributes failure to attain goals to personal inadequacies*

❏ *Individual's perceived loss of self-esteem results in cluster of affective, behavioral, and cognitive responses*

2. At least 20% of adult cancer patients have clinically significant depression during course of disease

3. Defining characteristics of depression must

❏ *Indicate a change from previous functioning*

❏ *Be persistent*

❏ *Occur for most of day*

❏ *Occur more days than not*

❏ *Be present for at least 2 weeks*

❏ *Include*

  ☐ Expressions of hopelessness, despair

  ☐ Inability to concentrate

  ☐ Change in physical activities, eating, sleeping, sexual activity

  ☐ Lowered self-esteem

  ☐ Feelings of failure

  ☐ Withdrawal from others

  ☐ Threats or attempts to commit suicide

  ☐ Suspicion and sensitivity to words and actions of others

  ☐ Misdirected anger toward self

  ☐ General irritability

  ☐ Guilt feelings

  ☐ Dependency on others

4. Treatment includes

❏ *Identification of stimuli that have resulted in loss of self-esteem*

❏ *Referral to another member of health care team if patient presents with longstanding history of depression*

- ❏ *Assisting patient to acknowledge feelings of hopelessness and despair by giving permission to discuss feelings through*
  - ☐ Attentive listening
  - ☐ Acknowledgment of feeling
  - ☐ Exploration of methods to deal positively with feelings
- ❏ *Assisting patient to focus on immediate goals of care to reduce overwhelming feelings of powerlessness*
- ❏ *Focusing on positive abilities of patient, contracting short-term goals of care*

■ Hopelessness

1. **Defined as subjective state in which individual sees limited or no alternatives or personal choices available and is unable to mobilize energy on own behalf**

2. **Characterized by**
   - ❏ *Passivity*
   - ❏ *Decreased verbalization*
   - ❏ *Flat affect*
   - ❏ *Verbalization of despondent or hopeless content*
   - ❏ *Lack of initiative*
   - ❏ *Decreased response to stimuli*
   - ❏ *Lack of involvement in care*
   - ❏ *Turning away from speaker*

❏ *Decreased appetite*

❏ *Increased sleep*

3. **Interventions include**

❏ *Assisting with reality surveillance*

☐ Review changes in and current health status

☐ Seek perceptions of patient with respect to health

☐ Confirm accurate perception

☐ Correct misconceptions of reality

☐ Encourage patient to discuss reality with others in same situation

❏ *Reinforcing personal power and ability*

☐ Review perceived strengths of patient and family

☐ Include patient in planning care, goals, schedule

☐ Encourage review of past successes in stressful times

☐ Reward approximations of goals

☐ Encourage value of use of needed external resources

❏ *Encouraging supportive relationships*

☐ Review number, types, and availability of supportive relationships

☐ Assist in helping patient to ask for support

☐ Encourage patient to continue contacts with supportive people

☐ Respect relationship of patient to higher being

☐ Encourage patient to express faith, if applicable

❏ *Creating future perspective*
  ☐ Review past occasions for hope
  ☐ Discuss meaning of hope from patient's perspective
  ☐ Establish short-term goals with patient and family
  ☐ Evaluate progress in achieving goals on routine basis
  ☐ Encourage expressions of hope for future

▮ Altered sexual health

1. **Defined as inability to express one's sexuality consistent with personal needs and preferences**

2. **Sexual health of people with cancer threatened by the sequelae associated with radical surgery, radiation, chemotherapy, and biotherapy**

3. **Characterized by**
  ❏ *Verbalizations of problems in sexuality*
  ❏ *Alterations in achieving perceived sex role*
  ❏ *Actual or perceived limitation imposed by disease or therapy*
  ❏ *Conflicts involving values*
  ❏ *Alteration in achieving sexual satisfaction*
  ❏ *Inability to achieve desired sexual satisfaction*
  ❏ *Frequent seeking of confirmation of desirability*

❏ *Alteration in relationship with significant other*

❏ *Change of interest in self and others*

4. **Interventions include**

❏ *Legitimizing patient's sexual concerns*

❏ *Encouraging patient to express sexual concerns with partner and health care team*

❏ *Providing anticipatory guidance with respect to sexual concerns*

❏ *Providing information needed for rehabilitation*

❏ *Discussing coping skills for changes experienced in communication, roles, relationships*

❏ *Helping patient to modify behaviors to accommodate limitations imposed by cancer or treatment*

❏ *Referring patient to professional therapist*

Social and Family Responses to Stress of Cancer

■ **Overview**

1. **Supportive relationships at home and in community assist individual responses to stress**

2. Family of origin or choice is most important social support for individual

3. Nurse's personal definitions of family or family values may vary from those of patients

4. Diagnosis of cancer precipitates significant changes for individual, members of family unit, and community

5. Responses vary among family members, across developmental stages of family, and with respect to economic and psychosocial resources

■ Psychosocial problems experienced by family members

1. Impaired relationships with family or significant others, or both

2. Impaired relationships with health care providers

3. Somatic side effects of disease and treatment

4. Difficulties in compliance with treatment

5. Mood disturbances

6. Difficulties in family roles

7. Difficulties in self-management

8. Financial difficulties

9. Transportation difficulties

10. Equipment difficulties

11. Significant concerns about body image

12. Denial

13. Cognitive impairment

■ Needs of family

1. Information

❏ *Family has assumed more responsibility in care of patient because of increased use of home health care services, outpatient care, and hospice services*

❏ *Families need to be taught how to administer care and where to find appropriate resources*

2. Communication

❏ *Communication becomes primary issue among family members as caregiving demands increase*

❏ *As demands of care increase, mood disturbances among family members, particularly anxiety and depression, become more prominent*

❏ *Communication patterns between patient and spouse, and between parents and children are strained*

❏ *Nurse plays important role in facilitating communication among family members via*
  □ One-on-one counselling
  □ Group sessions on communication
  □ Role modeling of facilitative communication
  □ Role-playing communications with individual family members

3. Coping skills

- ❏ *Modifying roles and relationship rules within family to meet demands imposed by illness*

- ❏ *Seeking help from outside sources*

- ❏ *Mobilizing action within household family*

4. Support services

- ❏ *Type, amount, and usage of support systems and services needed by caregivers of differing age, sex, and socioeconomic status is concern for health care providers*

- ❏ *Support services include*
  - ☐ Home management
  - ☐ Financial counselling
  - ☐ Anticipatory guidance
  - ☐ Transportation
  - ☐ Child care

- ❏ *Families have difficulty knowing where to go to get needed resources, and often have difficulty asking for help*

- ❏ *Nurses can help families identify and access support by*
  - ☐ Role-playing how to ask for help
  - ☐ Making list of tasks to be done
  - ☐ Giving extended family and friends opportunity to help, being specific about type and amount of help needed
  - ☐ Communicating needs via
    - ▪ Church newsletter or bulletins
    - ▪ Community newsletters or papers

- Handwritten, duplicated updates on how things are going to all supporters
- Development of telephone tree

Professional Responses to Cancer

■ Distancing

1. **Unconscious response of professionals, especially to people who are dying by**
   - ❏ *Delays in answering call lights*
   - ❏ *Infrequent visits*
   - ❏ *Failure to communicate*
   - ❏ *Maintaining "professionalism" in highly emotional situations*

2. **Especially prevalent when patient is not told truth**

3. **Enhances loneliness and fear of seriously ill**

4. **Showing genuine concern, being flexible and being good listener lessen professional distancing**

5. **Through communication strategies, nurses with high levels of interpersonal competence effect behavioral changes, comfort, establish and maintain relationships, create positive self-image for patient, and relay information**

6. **Nurses can enhance interpersonal skills by**
   Audiotaping and videotaping for feedback

❏ *Studying the literature to learn communication strategies*

❏ *Attending multidisciplinary conferences dealing with psychosocial needs of patients and families*

Caring

1. **Process that helps person attain or maintain health or peaceful death**

2. **Action-oriented and its intent is helpful**

3. **Moral commitment to protect human dignity**

4. **Begins with interest in another**

5. **Expands through knowledge and becomes commitment to help person to exist and to grow**

6. **Patients define caring behaviors among nurses as**

   ❏ *Physical care that is humane (considerate, competent, gentle, timely, and accessible)*

   ❏ *Emotional care that includes concern, involvement, sharing, touching (when culturally condoned), voluntary presence, and humor*

7. **Potentially negative outcomes of caring by nurses are overinvolvement and burnout**

Self-Care as Desired Psychosocial Outcomes

◼ **Includes attempts of individual to**

1. **Promote optimal health**
2. **Prevent illness**
3. **Detect symptoms**
4. **Manage chronic illness**

◼ **Is culturally specific**

◼ **Processes for achieving these goals include**

1. **Selecting healthy lifestyles**
2. **Self-monitoring and assessing symptoms**
3. **Perceiving and assigning meaning to symptoms**
4. **Evaluating severity of situation**
5. **Determining treatment alternatives**

◼ **Outcomes of self-care behaviors**

1. **Reduction in morbidity associated with illness**
2. **Increased use of health resources**
3. **Lowered cost of health care**
4. **More effective coping strategies**
5. **Enhanced role performance**

6. **Increased independence in health-related activities or activities of daily living, or both**

7. **Increased frequency of health promotion behaviors**

8. **Enhanced self-esteem and well-being**

Suggested Readings

1. McGee RF: Overview: Psychosocial aspects of cancer. In Groenwald SG, Frogge MH, Goodman M, Yarbro CH (eds.): *Cancer Nursing: Principles and Practice.* Boston: Jones and Bartlett, 1993, pp. 437–448.

2. Dorsett DS: The trajectory of cancer recovery. *Scholar Inq Nurs Prac* 5:175–184, 1991.

3. Clark J: Psychosocial responses of the patient. In Groenwald SL, Frogge MH, Goodman M, Yarbro CH (eds.): *Cancer Nursing: Principles and Practice.* Boston: Jones and Bartlett, 1993, pp. 449–467.

4. Clark J: Psychosocial responses of the family. In Groenwald SL, Frogge MH, Goodman M, Yarbro CH (eds.): *Cancer Nursing: Principles and Practice.* Boston: Jones and Bartlett, 1993, pp. 468–483.

▪ 14 ▪

Psychosocial Issues of Long-term Survival from Adult Cancer

Overview

◼ Early detection and effective multimodal therapies have increased significantly numbers of cancer survivors

◼ Cancer now considered chronic, life-threatening illness rather than terminal disease

◼ In the mid-1990s, over 8 million Americans had histories of cancer, with 4 million surviving 5 years or more

◼ Cancers with high and increasing 5-year survival rate include testicular cancer, colon cancer, cutaneous melanoma, breast cancer, Hodgkin's disease, prostate cancer, cervical cancer

◼ Cancer survivorship

1. Is experience of living through or beyond illness

2. Is a process, not a stage or component of survival

3. Requires consideration of cancer control rather than cure

■ "Seasons" or stages of survivorship include

1. **Acute stage**
   ❑ *Begins at diagnosis*
   ❑ *Deals with immediate effects of therapy*

2. **Extended stage**
   ❑ *Begins when disease is in remission or survivor has finished primary treatment course and starts consolidation or adjuvant therapy*

3. **Permanent stage**
   ❑ *Most frequently associated with "cure"*
   ❑ *Evolves from period of time when cancer activity or chance of its return markedly decreases, and disease is arrested permanently*

Critical Concerns of Cancer Survivors

■ Resources for food, shelter, medical care

1. Limited finances

2. Loss of job benefits

3. Lack of adequate follow-up medical care

■ **Physical attractiveness, fitness, physical function**

1. Any body image alteration
2. Energy reserve impairment
3. Residual physical disability

■ **Self-respect, integrity, autonomy**

1. Self-blame
2. Dependency
3. Self-doubt
4. Change from precancer lifestyle

■ **Intimate relationships**

1. Fears about hereditary transmission
2. Family stress related to illness
3. Alterations in customary social support
4. Sexual dysfunction
5. Concern about disclosure

■ **Social relationships**

1. Shunning and isolationism
2. Discriminatory practices
3. Concern about disclosure

■ **Recreation and play**

1. Physical compromise
2. Financial constraints
3. Fear of distancing self from health care team

■ Future

1. Fears of relapse and death
2. Dependence on health care providers
3. Survivor guilt
4. Uncertainty
5. Effects on family

Employment and Insurance Discrimination

■ Employment problems

1. **Employment problems are attributed to three myths about cancer**
   - ❏ *Cancer is a death sentence*
   - ❏ *Cancer is contagious*
   - ❏ *Cancer survivors are an unproductive drain on economy*

2. **Statistics indicate that**
   - ❏ *More than half of all Americans diagnosed with cancer will survive their illness*
   - ❏ *Cancer is not contagious*
   - ❏ *Cancer survivors have productivity rates similar to those of other workers*

3. **Employment-related problems include**
   - ❏ *Dismissal, demotion, and reduction or elimination of work-related benefits*

❑ *Situations arising from co-workers' attitudes about cancer*

❑ *Problems related to survivors' attitudes about how they should be perceived by others in workplace*

4. **Federal and state laws prohibit employment discrimination against qualified individuals with history of cancer**

■ **Insurance problems**

1. **25% to 30% of cancer survivors experience some form of insurance discrimination**

2. **Barriers to insurability include**
   ❑ *Refusal of new applications*
   ❑ *Policy cancellations or reductions*
   ❑ *Higher premiums*
   ❑ *Waived or excluded preexisting conditions*
   ❑ *Extended waiting periods*

3. **Insurance resources include**
   ❑ *Local or state insurance department*
   ❑ *Social security*
   ❑ *Medicare, Medicaid*
   ❑ *Group insurance plans*
   ❑ *Open enrollment periods*
   ❑ *Survivor organizations*
   ❑ *High-risk pools where available*

Suggested Readings

1. Leigh S, Boyle DMc, Loescher LJ, et al: Psychosocial issues of long-term survival from adult cancer. In Groenwald SL, Frogge MH, Goodman M, Yarbro CH (eds.): *Cancer Nursing: Principles and Practice* (3rd ed.). Boston: Jones and Bartlett, 1993, pp. 484–495.

2. Loescher LJ, Welch-McCaffrey D, Leigh SA, et al: Surviving adult cancer. *Ann Intern Med* 3:Part I: 411–432; Part II: 517–524, 1989.

3. Loescher LJ, Clark L, Atwood JR, et al: The impact of the cancer experience on long-term survivors. *Oncol Nurs Forum* 17:223–229, 1990.

4. Rowland JH: Survivorship: Beyond just a movement. *Cancer Invest* 9:607–608, 1991.

5. Quigley KM: The adult cancer survivor: Psychosocial consequences of cure. *Semin Oncol Nurs* 5:63–69, 1989.

PART IV

Manifestations of Cancer and Its Treatment

Bleeding Disorders

Overview

■ Bleeding is one of the most serious, potentially life-threatening problems for the person with cancer

■ Minor bleeding may be presenting symptom of cancer

■ Severe bleeding may indicate onset of progressive disease

■ Causes of bleeding in cancer

1. **Tumor factors**

   ❏ *Blood vessel invasion, erosion, and subsequent rupture*

   ❏ *Ulcerative effects of local infections at vessel sites*

   ❏ *Invasion and replacement of bone marrow by tumor*

2. Platelet abnormalities

❏ *Quantitative abnormalities*

  ☐ Thrombocytosis

  - Disorder involving increased number of circulating platelets (400,000–600,000 cells/mm^3)

  - Associated with chronic granulocytic anemia, and cancers of lung, ovary, pancreas, breast, kidney, and gastrointestinal tract

  - Venous thrombosis can occur, especially in patients with platelet counts greater than 1 million cells/mm^3

  ☐ Thrombocytopenia

  - Disorder involving reduction in number of circulating platelets

  - May be due to

    Decreased platelet production caused by tumor invasion of bone marrow or to acute or delayed effect of chemotherapy or radiotherapy

    Ninety percent of platelet production can be sequestered in spleen in patients with hypersplenism; thus, platelets are unavailable in circulation

    Idiopathic thrombocytopenia purpura can result in antibodies being formed against individual's own platelets

    Rapid replacement of intravascular volume of stored platelet-poor blood dilutes thrombocytes already present

Platelet function decreases due to decreased adhesiveness and decreased aggregation (e.g., with aspirin and nonsteroidal anti-inflammatory drugs [NSAIDs])

❏ *Qualitative abnormalities*
  ☐ Platelet malfunction
    ▪ Bleeding occurs despite normal platelet counts and coagulation factors
    ▪ May be due to malignancy itself or to partial release of platelet contents after contact with malignant tissue
    ▪ Many drugs also decrease platelet function (e.g., aspirin, NSAIDs, beta-lactam antibiotics, psychotropic drugs, some chemotherapeutic agents)

❏ *Hypocoagulation*
  ☐ Risk factors
    ▪ Tumor load
    ▪ Liver disease
    ▪ Vitamin K deficiency
    ▪ Excessive frozen plasma transfusions

❏ *Hypercoagulation*
  ☐ Disseminated intravascular coagulopathy (DIC) is most commonly caused by
    ▪ Infection
    ▪ Tumor
    ▪ Liver disease
    ▪ Intravascular hemorrhage
  ☐ Coagulation mechanism is triggered inappropriately by underlying disease process with abnormal activation of thrombin, upsetting balance of hemostasis

Approaches to Care

■ Assessment

1. Comprehensive history for patient at risk for bleeding

❏ *Bleeding tendencies*

❏ *Family history of any bleeding abnormalities*

❏ *Drugs and chemicals that interfere with coagulation*

❏ *General performance status*

❏ *Current blood component therapy*

❏ *Nutritional status; i.e., vitamin K or vitamin C deficiency*

❏ *Anemia*

2. Physical examination

❏ *Integumentary system*

☐ Bruising

☐ Petechiae

☐ Purpura

☐ Ecchymosis

☐ Acrocyanosis

☐ Oozing from venipuncture sites or injections, biopsy sites, central lines, catheters, or nasogastric tubes

❏ *Eyes and ears*

☐ Visual disturbances
☐ Periorbital edema
☐ Subconjunctival hemorrhage

- ☐ Headache
- ☐ Ear pain

❏ *Nose, mouth, and throat*
- ☐ Petechiae on nasal or oral mucosa
- ☐ Epistaxis
- ☐ Tenderness or bleeding from gums or oral mucosa

❏ *Cardiopulmonary system*
- ☐ Crackles
- ☐ Wheezes
- ☐ Stridor
- ☐ Dyspnea
- ☐ Tachypnea
- ☐ Cyanosis
- ☐ Hemoptysis
- ☐ Changes in vital signs
- ☐ Color and temperature of all extremities
- ☐ Peripheral pulses

❏ *Genitourinary system*
- ☐ Bleeding
- ☐ Character and amount of menses
- ☐ Urinary output

❏ *Musculoskeletal system*
- ☐ Bleeding into joints

❏ *Central nervous system*
- ☐ Mental status changes
  - Restlessness
  - Confusion
  - Lethargy
  - Dizziness
  - Obtundation
  - Seizures
  - Coma

3. Screening tests

- ❏ *Bleeding time*
- ❏ *Platelet count*
- ❏ *Whole-blood clot retraction test*
- ❏ *Prothrombin time*
- ❏ *Partial thromboplastin time*
- ❏ *Fibrin degradation products (FDP) test*

4. Manifestations

- ❏ *Internal bleeding may present as*
  - ☐ Massive hemoptysis
  - ☐ Severe hematemesis
  - ☐ Vaginal hemorrhage
  - ☐ Loss of consciousness
  - ☐ Hypovolemic shock

- ❏ *Loss of 6 to 8 cc of blood per day will precipitate iron-deficiency anemia*
  - ☐ Diagnostic indications of iron-deficiency anemia
    - ▪ Absence of stainable iron levels
    - ▪ Diminished plasma iron levels
    - ▪ Increased level of unsaturated iron-binding capacity
    - ▪ Reduced serum ferritin level
  - ☐ Symptoms of anemia
    - ▪ Fatigue
    - ▪ Weakness
    - ▪ Irritability
    - ▪ Dyspnea
    - ▪ Tachycardia

- ❏ *Clinical evidence of DIC*
  - ☐ Easy and spontaneous bleeding
  - ☐ Minor coagulation disorders or overt bleeding
  - ☐ Prolonged prothrombin time
  - ☐ Prolonged partial thromboplastin time

☐ Decreased platelet count
☐ Increased FDP

▨ Interventions

1. General bleeding

❑ *Direct and steady pressure to site of bleeding*

❑ *Mechanical pressure if bleeding site is not directly accessible*

❑ *Prophylactic arterial ligation*

❑ *Blood transfusions restore circulatory volume and oxygen-carrying capacity*

❑ *Oral or parenteral iron supplements may be indicated*

❑ *Human erythropoietin may stimulate erythropoiesis*

2. Thrombocytosis

❑ Thrombocytapheresis: *Rapidly removes large numbers of platelets*

❑ Marrow suppressive therapy: *Alkylating agents may be used to suppress hyperproliferative marrow*

❑ Radiation therapy: *Radioactive phosphorous may suppress hyperproliferative marrow*

3. Thrombocytopenia

❑ *Platelet transfusions*
❑ *Provide safe environment*
❑ *Minimal use of aspirin and NSAIDs*
❑ *Treatment of primary disease*

4. Hypocoagulation

- ❏ *Effective tumor therapy*
- ❏ *Plasma and plasma derivative therapy*
- ❏ *Albumin transfusions*
- ❏ *Plasma component therapy*
- ❏ *Parenteral vitamin K*

5. Hypercoagulation

- ❏ *Treatment of precipitating cause (i.e., sepsis or tumor)*
- ❏ *Heparin therapy may be useful for chronic DIC by inhibiting formation of new clots*
- ❏ *ε-aminocaproic acid (Amicar) is a fibrinolytic inhibitor and useful in management of DIC*
- ❏ *Blood replacement therapy*

6. Nursing interventions for persons at risk for or experiencing bleeding

- ❏ *Provide for person's physical safety*
- ❏ *Maintain person's skin integrity*
- ❏ *Apply pressure to injection sites*
- ❏ *Consider pharmacologic suppression of menses*
- ❏ *Instruct patient to avoid forceful coughing, sneezing, or nose blowing*
- ❏ *Provide for liberal use of stool softeners and laxatives*

7. Blood component therapy

- ❏ *Anemia*
  - ☐ Transfusions indicated when patient is short of breath

- □ One unit of packed red blood cells raises hematocrit by 3% and hemoglobin by 1 g/dl
- □ Patients who are prone to transfusion reactions require leukocyte-poor blood component therapy
- □ Plasma component therapy is administered for severe bleeding and shock
- □ All blood products given to a severely immunocompromised host should be irradiated to prevent lymphocyte engraftment

❏ *Thrombocytopenia*
  - □ Platelet transfusions are required when patient is at risk for bleeding or when bleeding occurs in presence of low platelets
  - □ One unit of platelets increases peripheral blood platelet level by 10,000 to 12,000 cells/mm^3
  - □ Goal is to maintain platelet count above 20,000 cells/mm^3 to prevent spontaneous bleeding
  - □ Failure to maintain an adequate platelet count is often due to infection, fever, DIC, or splenomegaly
  - □ Fever caused by platelets may be prevented by premedicating with antipyretics, corticosteroids, and/or antihistamines; meperidine may be given if patient is having shaking chills
  - □ Repeated exposure to human lymphocyte antigens (HLAs) on donor platelets may result in ineffective platelet therapy requiring HLA-matched or leukocyte-poor transfusions

- ❑ *Transfusion complications include*
  - ☐ Hemolytic and nonhemolytic transfusion reactions
  - ☐ Transmission of diseases
  - ☐ Graft-versus-host disease (in patients who had bone marrow transplantation)

- ❑ Home transfusion therapy: *Basic criteria include*
  - ☐ Physical limitations of patient that make travel difficult
  - ☐ Stable cardiopulmonary status
  - ☐ Absence of reactions to most recent transfusion
  - ☐ Cooperation on part of patient
  - ☐ Presence of responsible adult during and after transfusion
  - ☐ Telephone available for medical needs

Suggested Readings

1. Gobel BH: Bleeding disorders. In Groenwald S, Frogge M, Goodman M, and Yarbro CH (eds.): *Cancer Nursing: Principles and Practice* (3rd ed.). Boston: Jones and Bartlett, 1993, pp. 575–605.

2. Haeuber D, Spross JA: Alterations in protective mechanisms: Hematopoiesis and bone marrow depression. In Baird SB, McCorkle R, Grant M (eds.): *Cancer Nursing: A Comprehensive Textbook.* Philadelphia: WB Saunders, 1991, pp. 759–781.

3. Bagby GC, Segal GM: Growth factors and the control of hematopoiesis. In Hoffman R, Benz EJ, Shattil SJ, et al (eds.): *Hematology: Basic Principles and Practice.* New York: Churchill-Livingstone, 1991, pp. 97–121.

4. Feinstein DI: Treatment of disseminated intravascular coagulation. *Semin Thromb Hemost* 14:339–348, 1988.

5. Pisciotto PT (ed.): *Blood Transfusion Therapy: A Physician's Handbook* (3rd ed.). Arlington, VA: American Association of Blood Banks, 1989.

6. Rutman R, Kakaiya P, Miller WV: Home transfusion for the cancer patient. *Semin Oncol Nurs* 6:163–167, 1990.

▪ 16 ▪
Cardiac Tamponade

Overview: Cardiac Tamponade

- ▪ Occurs when excessive fluid accumulates in pericardial space

- ▪ Excess fluid severely compromises heart, resulting in

1. Disruption in pressure gradients
2. Decreased diastolic filling
3. Decreased stroke volume and cardiac output

- ▪ Both cancer and cancer therapy can initiate cardiac tamponade

- ▪ Neoplastic involvement of heart is rarely diagnosed before patient dies

- ▪ About 3% of cancer patients develop cardiac tamponade

■ Pericardial effusion and constrictive pericarditis can be caused by tumors that have metastasized to pericardium or have directly extended into pericardium

■ Radiation therapy to mediastinum can damage pericardium, causing constrictive pericarditis

■ Rate of fluid accumulation, compliance of pericardium, myocardial size, and intravascular volume affect rate of onset and severity of pericardial effusion

■ Tumors most commonly involved are

1. Lung
2. Breast
3. Leukemia
4. Hodgkin's disease
5. Lymphoma
6. Melanoma
7. Gastrointestinal cancer
8. Sarcoma

Approaches to Care

■ Assessment
1. Clinical manifestations
   ❑ Increased heart rate
   ❑ Peripheral vasoconstriction

❏ *Water and sodium retention*

❏ *Early symptoms and signs*
   □ Weakness
   □ Retrosternal chest pain
   □ Shortness of breath
   □ Venous distention
   □ Distant heart sounds
   □ Paradoxical pulse

❏ *Late symptoms and signs*
   □ Hypotension
   □ Tachycardia
   □ Diminished arterial pulse
   □ Cough
   □ Peripheral edema
   □ Diaphoresis
   □ Abdominal distention, nausea, vomiting
   □ Confusion
   □ Cyanosis

2. Diagnostic measures

❏ *Echocardiogram is easiest and most sensitive tool*

❏ *Computed tomographic scan to estimate volume of effusion and thickness of pericardium*

❏ *Chest x-ray film reveals enlarged, globular, bottle-shaped heart*

■ Treatment

1. Supportive therapy, initiated immediately, includes

❏ *Volume expanders*
❏ *Fresh-frozen plasma*

❏ *Vasoactive agents*
❏ *Oxygen*

2. Pericardiocentesis

❏ *Is performed if "rule of 20" is present*
   ☐ Central venous pressure greater than 20 mm Hg
   ☐ Paradoxical pulse greater than 20 mm Hg
   ☐ Pulse pressure less than 20 mm Hg

❏ *Performed under echocardiographic guidance*

❏ *Fluid is sent for cytologic study to determine most appropriate cancer therapy*

3. Permanent resolution occurs through systemic therapy or local treatment of cancer

4. Further palliation of effusion may be obtained through surgical interventions

❏ *Subxiphoid pericardiotomy, or pericardial window*

❏ *Pleuropericardial window*

❏ *Total pericardiectomy*

5. Potential surgical complications

❏ *Infection*   ❏ *Pleural effusion*
❏ *Arrhythmias*   ❏ *Pneumothorax*
❏ *Bleeding*   ❏ *Costochondritis*
❏ *Atelectasis*

6. Sclerosing therapy is effective in about 50% of attempts

❏ *Agents used are tetracycline, quinacrine, thiotepa, nitrogen mustard, and 5-fluorouracil*

❏ *Transient chest pain, fever, nausea, and arrhythmias may result*

7. **Intrapericardial infusion of cytotoxic agents may be performed; cisplatin has most often been used (10 mg in 50 ml normal saline for 5 days)**

8. **Corticosteroids can help alleviate inflammation of constrictive pericarditis**

9. **Radiation therapy has been used to treat extremely radiosensitive tumors**

10. **Unsuccessful resolution can severely debilitate person or result in death**

11. **If effusion is chronic condition, limited outlook for survival exists**

12. **Supportive terminal care is usually needed**

Suggested Readings

1. Dietz KA, Flaherty AM: Oncologic emergencies. In Groenwald SL, Frogge MH, Goodman M, Yarbro CH (eds.): *Cancer Nursing: Principles and Practice* (3rd ed.). Boston: Jones and Bartlett, 1993, 813–816.

2. Helms SR, Carlson MD: Cardiovascular emergencies. *Semin Oncol* 16(6):463–470, 1989.

3. Joiner GA: Neoplastic cardiac tamponade. *Crit Care Nurs* 11(2):50–58, 1991.

4. Press OW, Livingston R: Management of malignant pericardial effusion and tamponade. *JAMA* 257:1088–1092, 1987.

▪ 17 ▪
Disseminated Intravascular Coagulation

Overview: Disseminated Intravascular Coagulation (DIC)

■ Characterized by widespread clotting within arterioles and capillaries and simultaneous hemorrhage

■ Occurs in fewer than 15% of persons with cancer

■ Associated conditions include

1. Intravascular hemolysis

2. Bacteremia (gm + or gm −)

3. Viremia (cytomegalovirus, hepatitis, varicella)

4. Mucin-producing adenocarcinomas (gastric, lung, pancreas, prostate)

5. **Hematologic malignancy (leukemia, lymphoma)**

6. **Implanted devices**

7. **Liver disease**

■ **Microvascular thrombosis and bleeding from multiple sites occur simultaneously with DIC**

1. **Fibrinogen is consumed by thrombin-induced clotting and plasmin-induced fibrinolysis**

2. **Decreased macrophage-clearing function limits removal of activated clotting factors**

3. **Rapid coagulation exceeds ability of liver to clear fibrin split products (FSPs)**

4. **Excess FSPs inhibit clotting**

5. **Consumable factors I, II, V, VIII are depleted by microvascular clotting**

Approaches to Care

■ **Assessment**

1. **Clinical manifestations**

❑ *Early symptoms and signs*
   ☐ Anxiety, restlessness
   ☐ Tachycardia, tachypnea
   ☐ Headache
   ☐ Conjunctival hemorrhage
   ☐ Periorbital petechiae
   ☐ Oozing blood
   ☐ Bleeding gums

❑ *Late symptoms and signs*
  - ☐ Change in mentation
  - ☐ Joint pain
  - ☐ Tarry stool, melena
  - ☐ Frank hematuria
  - ☐ Hemoptysis

2. **Diagnostic measures**

❑ *DIC is defined by the presence of two or more of the following abnormalities*

  - ☐ Prothrombin time 3 seconds or more greater than control

  - ☐ Activated partial thromboplastin time 5 or more seconds greater than control

  - ☐ Thrombin time prolonged by 3 or more seconds more than control

  - ☐ Fibrinogen less than 150 mg/dl

  - ☐ Fibrin split products equal to or greater than 40 mcg/ml

  - ☐ Decreased platelet count

■ **Treatment**

1. **Only effective intervention is treatment of underlying malignancy; all other measures are only supportive**

2. **Give platelets and fresh-frozen plasma to replace consumed blood components**

3. **Give fresh-frozen plasma and antithrombin III concentrate to neutralize excess thrombin and slow DIC process**

4. **Administer heparin (7.5 U/kg/hr) as continuous infusion to avoid peaks in effect**

❏ *Inhibits factors IX and X to halt clotting cascade*

❏ *Contraindicated if there is excessive bleeding in closed space, because vital functions could be compromised*

❏ *Stopped immediately if person complains of headache or displays signs of frank bleeding*

❏ *Considered controversial therapy*

5. **Give ε-aminocaproic acid in conjunction with heparin to maintain platelet and fibrinogen levels**

❏ *Controversial*

❏ *Not used in most cases since inhibition of fibrinolytic system can lead to widespread fibrin deposition in microcirculation*

6. **Monitor vital signs, urine output, and blood loss**

7. **Maintain quiet environment**

8. **Give medications to suppress symptoms (e.g., cough, vomiting) that will increase intracranial pressure**

9. **Initiate bleeding precautions**

10. **Monitor for signs of cardiogenic shock: hypovolemia, hypoxia, hypotension, oliguria**

11. **Effective control of DIC is measured by normal coagulation screen and platelet count**

12. **Nursing measures**

❑ *Reduce potential for injury*
❑ *Enhance tissue perfusion*
❑ *Educate patient regarding early signs*

Suggested Readings

1. Dietz KA, Flaherty AM: Oncologic emergencies. In Groenwald SL, Frogge MH, Goodman M, Yarbro CH (eds.): *Cancer Nursing: Principles and Practice* (3rd ed.). Boston: Jones and Bartlett, 1993, pp. 805–810.

2. Rooney A, Haviley C: Nursing management of disseminated intravascular coagulation. *Oncol Nurs Forum* 12:15–22, 1985.

3. Bell TN: Disseminated intravascular coagulation and shock. *Crit Care Nurs Clin North Am* 2:255–268, 1990.

4. Young LM: DIC: The insidious killer. *Crit Care Nurs* 10:26–33, 1990.

▪ 18 ▪
Fatigue

Overview

■ Definition

1. Fatigue is a complex concept associated with such terms as
   - ❏ *Tiredness*
   - ❏ *Exhaustion*
   - ❏ *Weariness*
   - ❏ *Drowsiness*
   - ❏ *Malaise*
   - ❏ *Weakness*
   - ❏ *Asthenia*
   - ❏ *Somnolence*
   - ❏ *Lack of energy*

2. Objective indicator of fatigue relates to person's ability to maintain specific activities

3. Subjective experience of fatigue relates to feeling state; it has voluntary component

■ Pathophysiology

1. *Acute fatigue* is an expected outcome of strenuous physical and mental activity and has same protective effect as acute pain

2. Fatigue in individuals with cancer

❑ *Does not respond to rest*

❑ *Persists over time*

❑ *Often interferes with performance of usual daily activities*

3. Cause of *chronic fatigue* in cancer has not been established, but is a combination of physical factors such as

❑ *Tumor burden*

❑ *Physical stress of treatment*

❑ *Environmental changes during hospitalization*

❑ *Psychologic factors such as fear of death*

❑ *Changes in social relationships and roles*

❑ *Nutritional changes*

❑ *Side effects of treatment*

❑ *Symptoms of disease*

❑ *Loss of sleep from side effects or symptoms of disease and psychologic factors such as*
   ☐ Anxiety   ☐ Depression

Approaches to Care

◼ Assessment

1. Patient describes problems associated with fatigue

2. **Nurse observes individual's**

   ❏ *Appearance*
   ❏ *Level of consciousness*
   ❏ *Activity level*

3. **Patient describes his or her current activities in comparison to usual daily activities**

4. **Nurse assesses patient's acceptance of limitations imposed by fatigue**

■ **Treatment interventions**

1. **Prepare patient in advance of treatment for what to expect in relation to fatigue**

2. **Plan for rest periods**

3. **Prioritize and rearrange patient's activities**

4. **Exercise helps relieve fatigue in some individuals**

5. **Manipulate patient's environment to allow undisturbed time for sleep and rest**

Suggested Readings

1. Nail LM, Winningham ML: Fatigue. In Groenwald SL, Frogge MH, Goodman M, Yarbro CH (eds.): *Cancer Nursing: Principles and Practice* (3rd ed.). Boston: Jones and Bartlett, 1993, pp. 608–619.

2. Irvine DM, Vincent L, Bubela N, et al: A critical appraisal of the research literature investigating fatigue in the individual with cancer. *Cancer Nurs* 14(4):188–199, 1991.

3. Blesch KS, Paice JA, Wickham R, et al: Correlates of fatigue in people with breast or lung cancer. *Oncol Nurs Forum* 18:81–87, 1991.

▪ 19 ▪
Hypercalcemia

Overview

▪ Occurs when level of serum calcium exceeds normal limits

▪ Untreated hypercalcemia can lead to life-threatening alterations of cardiac, neurologic, and renal function

▪ Most common life-threatening metabolic abnormality in cancer patients

▪ Occurs in 10% to 20% of persons with cancer and is severely underdiagnosed

▪ Occurrence heralds lack of control of malignant disease process

▪ Occurs as result of increased bone resorption caused by

1. Bone destruction by tumor invasion

2. Increased levels of parathyroid hormone, osteoclast-activating factor, or prostaglandin produced by tumor

■ **Risk factors**

1. **Primary tumors of breast, lung, kidney**
2. **Osteolytic bone lesions**
3. **Hematologic malignancies**
4. **Squamous cell lung cancer**
5. **Head and neck cancers**
6. **Hyperparathyroidism**
7. **Immobilization**
8. **Anorexia, nausea, vomiting**
9. **Renal failure**

■ **Humoral mediator factors involved include**

1. **Transforming growth factor**
2. **Interleukin 1**
3. **Tumor necrosis factor**
4. **Prostaglandin following hormone therapy**

Approaches to Care

■ **Assessment**

1. **Clinical manifestations relate to effects of excess calcium on smooth, skeletal, and cardiac muscle**

   ❑ Gastrointestinal: *Anorexia, nausea, vomiting, constipation, pain, dehydration*

   ❑ Neuromuscular: *Lethargy, confusion, stupor, convulsions, hyporeflexia*

❑ Cardiac: *Bradycardia, tachycardia, EKG changes (increased PR interval, decreased QT interval)*

❑ Renal: *Polyuria, polydypsia, decreased renal concentrating ability, renal insufficiency*

2. Diagnostic measures

❑ *Laboratory studies provide definitive diagnosis*

❑ *Three categories of hypercalcemia have been defined*

☐ Serum calcium level of 10.5 to 12.0 mg/dl and asymptomatic

☐ Serum calcium level of 12 to 13 mg/dl and asymptomatic

☐ Serum calcium level of 13 mg/dl or more and symptomatic

❑ *Serum calcium level must be "corrected" to be accurate. It can be calculated as:*

Corrected serum calcium = Measured serum calcium + (4.0 − serum albumin) × 0.8

■ Treatment

1. Tumor control is only long-term effective measure

2. Emergency intervention is needed if serum calcium level is greater than 13 mg/dl

3. Major focus of therapy

❑ *Vigorous hydration with 4 to 6 liters of normal saline per day to*

☐ Restore normal fluid volume

  □ Increase glomerular filtration
  □ Promote urinary calcium excretion

❏ *Parenteral furosemide 40 to 80 mg every 6 hours*

❏ *Monitor fluid and electrolyte balance closely*
  □ Vigorous hydration can lead to hypokalemia, hypocalcemia, and hypomagnesemia
  □ Blood urea nitrogen and creatinine are monitors of renal function

❏ *Give mithramycin intravenously, 15 to 25 μg/kg body weight to inhibit bone resorption*
  □ Decreases serum calcium within 12 hours
  □ Peak effect at 48 hours
  □ May cause nausea, vomiting, bone marrow suppression, and hepatic and renal changes
  □ Infiltration at intravenous site can cause necrosis

❏ *Calcitonin 4 Medical Research Council units/kg of body weight subcutaneously every 12 hours can inhibit bone resorption*
  □ Rapid effect, duration of response is limited
  □ Response limited to 24 to 72 hours
  □ Glucocorticoids are given to improve effect
  □ Risk of anaphylaxis

❏ *Use phosphate 75 mmol intravenously if other measures fail*
  □ Acts within minutes
  □ Danger of hypotension
  □ Hypocalcemia, renal failure can occur

- ❏ *Bisphosphonates are potent inhibitors of osteoclastic bone resorption*
  - ☐ Well-tolerated, minimal side effects
  - ☐ Two agents available in U.S.
    - ■ Etidronate (7.5 mg/kg/d intravenously)
    - ■ Pamidronate (30 mg intravenously)
  - ☐ Produce normocalcemia in 5 to 9 days
  - ☐ Duration of response is 2 to 4 weeks
- ❏ *Gallium nitrate effective in reducing serum calcium salts in bone*
  - ☐ Give 200 mg/m^2 in continuous intravenous infusion for 5 days
  - ☐ Produces normocalcemia in more than 80% of cases
- ❏ *Oral phosphate 1 to 3 mg three times a day can control chronic, mild hypercalcemia*
  - ☐ Diarrhea may be limiting side effect
  - ☐ Perianal care is important to prevent skin breakdown
  - ☐ Encourage patient to take sitz baths
- ❏ *Treatment of hypercalcemia is directly related to effectiveness of cancer control*

Suggested Readings

1. Dietz KA, Flaherty AM: Oncologic emergencies. In Groenwald SL, Frogge MH, Goodman M, Yarbro CH (eds.): *Cancer Nursing: Principles and Practice* (3rd ed.). Boston: Jones and Bartlett, 1993, pp. 816–821.

2. Mundy GR: Pathophysiology of cancer-associated hypercalcemia. *Semin Oncol* 17(suppl. 5):10–15, 1990.

3. Bajorunas DR: Clinical manifestations of cancer-related hypercalcemia. *Semin Oncol* 17(suppl. 5): 16–25, 1990.

4. Mahon SM: Signs and symptoms associated with malignancy-induced hypercalcemia. *Cancer Nurs* 12:153–160, 1989.

5. Heath D: The treatment of hypercalcemia of malignancy. *Clin Endocrinol* 34:155–157, 1991.

■ 20 ■
Infection

Overview

■ Major cause of morbidity and mortality

1. Implicated in 50% of cancer deaths from solid tumors

2. Implicated in 80% of deaths from leukemia

■ Risk factors

1. Abnormalities of immune system

2. Decreased polymorphonuclear neutrophils (PMNs)

3. Acquired immunodeficiency syndrome (AIDS)

4. Poor nutrition

5. Cancer therapies

■ **Common sites of infection are**

1. **Mouth and pharynx**
2. **Respiratory tract**
3. **Skin, soft tissue, intravascular catheters**
4. **Perineal region**
5. **Urinary tract**
6. **Nose and sinuses**
7. **Gastrointestinal (GI) tract**

■ **Types of infection and specific treatments**

1. **Bacteria**
   - ❏ *Gram-negative bacteria; e.g.,* Escherichia coli, Klebsiella pneumoniae, Pseudomonas aeruginosa

   - ❏ *Gram-positive bacteria; e.g.,* Staphylococcus aureus, Staphylococcus epidermidis

   - ❏ *Treatment begins immediately*
     - ☐ Immediate empiric antibiotic therapy
     - ☐ Highly specific therapy initiated once an organism is identified
     - ☐ Combination antibiotic therapy usually includes an aminoglycoside and penicillin and/or cephalosporin

2. **Mycobacteria**
   - ❏ *Less common*

   - ❏ *Usually associated with defects in cellular immunity*

❏ *Latent* Mycobacterium tuberculosis *may be reactivated*

❏ Mycobacterium avium-intracellulare *(MAI) is common with AIDS*

❏ *Treatment for tuberculosis is isoniazid*

❏ *Treatment for MAI is combination antibiotic therapy*

3. Fungi

❏ *Increasingly important cause of infections for cancer patients*

❏ *Contributing factors include*
   ☐ Prolonged granulocytopenia
   ☐ Implanted vascular access devices
   ☐ Administration of parenteral nutrition
   ☐ Corticosteroids
   ☐ Prolonged antibiotic usage

❏ Candida *is most common causative agent*

❏ Aspergillus, Cryptococcus, Histoplasma, Phycomycetes, Coccidioides *are common fungi*

❏ *Treatment is confounded by*
   ☐ Difficulty culturing organisms
   ☐ Limited number of effective agents

❏ *Amphotericin B is drug of choice*
   ☐ Side effects including fever, chills, rigors, nausea, vomiting, hypotension, bronchospasm, and seizures require intensive support
   ☐ Nephrotoxicity is the major toxicity

❏ *Flucytosine (5-FC), fluconazole, ketoconazole, and miconazole are also used*

4. Virus

❏ *Usually herpes simplex virus (HSV), varicella zoster virus (VZV), cytomegalovirus (CMV), and hepatitis A or B*

❏ *Acyclovir is drug of choice for HSV and VZV*

❏ *Vidarabine is effective if used early*

❏ *Ganciclovir and foscarnet are used for CMV*

5. Protozoa and parasites

❏ *Cause infections associated with defects in cell-mediated immunity*

❏ *Can be difficult to treat*

❏ *Can quickly become life-threatening*

❏ Pneumocystis carinii, Toxoplasma gondii, Cryptosporidium *are common*

❏ *Treatment of* P. carinii
  ☐ Trimethoprim-sulfamethoxazole, dapsone, or pentamidine
  ☐ High-risk patients (e.g., AIDS patients) are sometimes treated prophylactically

❏ *Treatment of* T. gondii
  ☐ Pyrimethamine plus sulfadiazine

❏ *No treatment is known for* Cryptosporidium

Approaches to Care

■ Prevention

1. Meticulous hand washing by caregivers

2. Avoidance of crowds and infected individuals

3. If granulocytopenia is present, invasive procedures should be avoided

4. Adequate nutrition

5. Meticulous personal hygiene

6. Avoiding skin trauma

■ Assessment

1. If number of circulating polymorphonuclear neutrophils (PMNs) is decreased, defenses are reduced

   ❑ *Absolute granulocyte count (AGC) is measure of risk*

   AGC = Total white blood cell count ×
   (% PMNs + % bands)

   ❑ *Individuals whose AGC is less than $1000/mm^3$ are granulocytopenic*

   ❑ *If AGC is less than $500/mm^3$, patient is severely granulocytopenic*

2. Culture from all potential sites of infection before giving antibiotics

3. Closely observe patient's response to therapy

4. **Monitor efficacy of treatment, vital signs, chest x-ray films, and laboratory data**

5. **Assess for signs of septic shock**
   - ❏ *Early shock*
     - ☐ Low-grade fever, possible shaking chill
     - ☐ Flushed, warm skin
     - ☐ Tachycardia, normal to slightly low blood pressure
     - ☐ Transient decrease in urine output
     - ☐ Hyperventilation
     - ☐ Alert, possible mild confusion, apprehension
     - ☐ Nausea, vomiting, diarrhea
   - ❏ *Late shock*
     - ☐ Febrile
     - ☐ Cold, clammy, acrocyanosis
     - ☐ Hypotension, decreased cardiac output, peripheral edema
     - ☐ Oliguria, anuria
     - ☐ Pulmonary edema
     - ☐ Restlessness, anxiety, confusion, lethargy, coma
     - ☐ Possible blood in stool or emesis

■ **Treatment of patient with granulocytopenia and fever**

1. **Empiric broad-spectrum antibiotic therapy**

2. **Isolation precautions and protected environment**

3. **Administration of colony-stimulating factors (granulocyte and granulocyte-macrophage)**

4. **Supportive care to maintain fluid and electrolyte levels, oxygen when needed, nutrition support**

■ **Treatment of patient with gram-negative sepsis**

1. **Septic shock develops in 27% to 46% of cases**

2. **Mortality can reach 80% unless aggressive therapy is initiated**

3. **Treatment measures to reverse shock and sepsis include**

   ❏ *Adequate oxygenation*

   ❏ *Effective circulation with fluid replacement and vasoactive agents*

   ❏ *Immediate broad-spectrum antibiotic therapy*

   ❏ *Observe for complications of sepsis: disseminated intravascular coagulation, renal failure, heart failure, GI ulcers, hepatic abnormalities*

■ **Nursing interventions**

1. **Practice meticulous hand washing and hygiene**

2. **Take appropriate protective measures and wear protective clothing**

3. **Ensure that patient has adequate fluid and dietary intake**

4. **Ensure that patient receives adequate rest**

5. **Use aseptic technique for invasive procedures**

6. **Avoid trauma, especially to skin**

7. **Culture suspicious areas**

8. **Avoid potential sources of infection**

Suggested Readings

1. Ellerhorst-Ryan J: Infection. In Groenwald SL, Frogge MH, Goodman M, Yarbro CH (eds.): *Cancer Nursing: Principles and Practice* (3rd ed.). Boston: Jones and Bartlett, 1993, pp. 557–574.

2. Workman ML: Inflammatory responses. In Workman ML, Ellerhorst-Ryan JM, Koertge VH (eds.): *Nursing Care of the Immunocompromised Patient.* Philadelphia: WB Saunders, 1993, pp. 14–31.

3. Shimpff SC: Infections in patients with cancer: Overview and epidemiology. In Moosa AR, Schimpff SC, Robson MC (eds.): *Comprehensive Textbook of Oncology,* Vol 2 (2nd ed.). Baltimore: Williams & Wilkins, 1991, pp. 1720–1732.

4. Brandt B: Nursing protocol for the patient with neutropenia. *Oncol Nurs Forum* 17(suppl. 1):9–15, 1990.

▪ 21 ▪
Integumentary Alterations

Overview

■ **Alterations to skin**

1. Radiotherapy

❏ *Major effect of radiation on dividing cells is cell death*

❏ *Radiosensitivity of cells varies*
   □ Cells with rapid turnover (e.g., skin cells, mucous membrane cells, hematopoietic stem cells) are radiosensitive
   □ Cells that do not divide regularly or at all (e.g., muscle cells, nerve cells) are radioresistant

❏ *Factors that determine degree, onset, and duration of radiation-induced skin reactions*
   □ *Equipment:* Energy or particular beam quality of machine influences surface or skin dose
   □ Bolus material on skin reduces skin-sparing effect of radiation therapy, allowing for maximum dose at level of skin

- ☐ Tangential field increases skin dose
- ☐ Concomitant chemotherapy enhances radiation effect
- ☐ Treatment of areas of skin apposition are prone to increased reactions secondary to warmth, moisture, and lack of aeration
- ☐ Epidermis thins with age, has diminished elasticity, and decreased dermal turgor resulting in delayed healing

2. Chemotherapy effects

❏ *Hyperpigmentation*
- ☐ Occurs in dark-skinned individuals
- ☐ Drugs
  - ▪ Cyclophosphamide
  - ▪ Doxorubicin
  - ▪ Methotrexate
  - ▪ 5-Fluorouracil

❏ *Hypersensitivity*
- ☐ *L-asparaginase:* Acute urticaria
- ☐ *Taxol:* Hypotension, rash, bradycardia, dyspnea
- ☐ *Cisplatin:* Pruritis, cough, dyspnea, angioedema, bronchospasm, rash, urticaria
- ☐ *Teniposide and etoposide:* Dyspnea, wheezing, hypotension, urticaria, pruritis, angioedema, facial flushing, and rash
- ☐ *Dactinomycin:* Folliculitis

❏ Acral erythema: *Intensely painful erythema, scaling, and epidermal sloughing from palms and soles followed by desquamation. Occurs with*
- ☐ Continuous infusions of 5-fluorouracil
- ☐ Doxorubicin
- ☐ High-dose cytarabine
- ☐ Floxuridine

❏ *Pruritis: Occurs in*
  ❏ Hodgkin's disease
  ❏ Multiple myeloma
  ❏ Aminoglutethimide
  ❏ Antibiotic reaction
  ❏ Radiation skin changes

❏ *Photosensitivity (enhanced skin response to ultraviolet radiation)*
  ❏ May present like sunburn with erythema, edema, blisters, hyperpigmentation, and desquamation or peeling
  ❏ Occurs following skin exposure to ultraviolet (UV) light with
    ▪ 5-Fluorouracil
    ▪ Dacarbazine
    ▪ Vinblastine
    ▪ High-dose methotrexate

❏ *Vesicant chemotherapy extravasation*
  ❏ Infiltration of chemotherapeutic agent (vesicant) that, if infiltrated, can cause blistering, pain, ulceration, necrosis, and sloughing of damaged tissue
  ❏ Occurs in 0.5% to 5.0% of patients receiving peripheral intravenous chemotherapy

3. Malignant wounds

❏ *Most often seen in patients with cancers of breast, stomach, lung, uterus, kidney, ovary, colon, and bladder, and melanoma, sarcoma, and lymphoma*

❏ *Poor vascular perfusion and altered collagen synthesis result in tissue ischemia and necrosis*

❏ *Mycosis fungoides is a T-cell lymphoma that can develop into fungating skin lesions*

■ Alterations to hair

1. Radiation effects

❏ *Extent and duration of radiation-induced alopecia depend on*
- ☐ Individual's normal hair growth rate
- ☐ Area being treated
- ☐ Dose per fraction
- ☐ Total dose delivered to area

❏ *Complete scalp hair loss is seen following whole-brain radiation*

❏ *Significant hair loss occurs after dose of 45 to 55 Gy*

❏ *Hair loss may be permanent if higher doses of radiation are given*

❏ *If hair regrows, it usually begins 8 to 9 weeks following completion of treatment*

2. Chemotherapy effects

❏ *Extent of hair loss depends on*
- ☐ Type of chemotherapy   ☐ Schedule
- ☐ Dose of drug

❏ *Drugs most commonly associated with alopecia*
- ☐ Bleomycin   ☐ Doxorubicin
- ☐ Cyclophosphamide   ☐ Vinblastine
- ☐ Dactinomycin   ☐ Taxol
- ☐ Daunorubicin

❏ *Hair loss occurs by*
  ◻ *Atrophy* of hair root. Hair falls out over 2 to 3 weeks
  ◻ *Partial atrophy* of hair bulb and narrowing of hair shaft that causes breakage

❏ *Hair loss is temporary*
  ◻ Regrowth is evident in 4 to 6 weeks after chemotherapy
  ◻ Hair returns to its normal color and texture in about 1 year

▉ Alterations of nails

1. Radiation to nails can result in decreased growth rates and development of ridges when nail attempts to grow

2. Chemotherapy causes

  ❏ Pigmentation *(with doxorubicin, 5-fluorouracil)*

  ❏ Beau's lines: *Transverse white lines or grooves*

  ❏ Onycholysis: *Partial nail separation seen with 5-fluorouracil, bleomycin, doxorubicin, taxol, and taxotere*

▉ Alterations of glands

1. Radiation to skin
  ❏ *Destruction of sebaceous glands*
  ❏ *Subsequent pruritis and inelasticity*

2. Complete and permanent destruction of sweat gland function occurs with skin dose greater than 30 Gy delivered in 3 weeks

Approaches to Care

◼ Skin

1. Radiation therapy

❏ *Assessment*

□ Assess condition of skin prior to treatment, weekly during treatment, 1 to 2 weeks following completion of treatment, and at each follow-up appointment thereafter

□ Consistency of assessment and documentation is imperative

□ Grading scales provide an objective system of categorizing impaired skin integrity

❏ *Clinical manifestations*

□ Acute skin reactions

▪ Occur weeks to months after first exposure

▪ Usually temporary

▪ Include erythema, dry desquamation, pruritis, hyperpigmentation, and moist desquamation

▪ Higher doses given over shorter periods of time to larger volumes of tissue result in more severe acute reactions

□ Late skin reactions

▪ Usually manifest months to years after exposure

▪ Usually permanent and often become more severe as time goes on

▪ Include photosensitivity, pigmentation changes, atrophy, fibrosis, telangiectasia, and, rarely, ulceration and necrosis

❏ *Interventions*

- ☐ Patient education prior to therapy to promote self-care behavior
  - Anticipated skin reactions
  - Onset and duration of reactions
  - Skin care guidelines to follow before and after radiation
- ☐ During treatment patient should
  - Shower or bathe using lukewarm water
  - Avoid harsh soap
  - Avoid ointments, creams, lotions, deodorant, perfume, cologne, powder, and cosmetics to skin
  - If instructed, apply recommended mild, water-soluble lubricant to reduce itching and discomfort
  - Avoid shaving treated areas if possible
  - Avoid extremes of temperature
  - Avoid tight-fitting clothing made of irritating fabric
  - Avoid exposing skin to sun
  - Avoid applying tape or adhesive bandages to skin in radiation treatment field
  - Drink at least 3 quarts of fluid each day
- ☐ Two to three weeks after treatment, patient should
  - Apply unscented hydrophilic emollient (lotion or cream) 2 to 3 times each day for 1 to 2 months after treatment and then daily

- Always avoid exposing previously irradiated skin to sun, or use sunscreen with sun protection factor (SPF) 15 or greater
- ☐ Severe acute radiation skin reactions
  - Dry desquamation with pruritis

    Increase frequency of lubricants, avoiding application 3 hours prior to treatment

    Apply cloths soaked in mild astringent to irritated area for 15 minutes 3 to 4 times a day

    Use mild topical steroids, avoiding application 3 hours prior to treatment
  - Moist desquamation

    Use mild astringent soaks as described above

    Apply hydrogel primary wound dressings, cover with nonadherent dressing, and secure with paper tape

    Apply occlusive hydrocolloid dressings

2. Chemotherapy

- ❏ *Cutaneous hypersensitivity*
  - ☐ Manifestations
    - Early manifestations are urticaria and angioedema
    - Hypotension, rash, dyspnea, and bronchospasm may occur within 10 minutes of initiating the drug
    - May progress to severe anaphylaxis
  - ☐ Treatment
    - Decrease infusion rate
    - Premedicate with antihistamines and steroids

❏ *Acral edema*
  □ Manifestations
    ■ Intensely painful erythema, scaling, and epidermal sloughing from the palms and soles
    ■ Followed by desquamation and reepithelialization of skin
  □ Treatment
    ■ Suspension of chemotherapy until symptoms have subsided
    ■ If symptoms recur, therapy may be discontinued

❏ *Pruritis*
  □ Assessment
    ■ For possible cause of itching and aggravating factors
    ■ Localization, onset, duration, and intensity of itching
    ■ Prior history of pruritis
    ■ Past or present cancer, cancer treatment, noncancer systemic disease, or use of analgesics or antibiotics
    ■ For presence of infection
  □ Treatment
    ■ Encourage adequate water intake
    ■ Suggest medicated baths to soothe
    ■ Apply local anesthetic creams
    ■ Encourage patient to employ alternate cutaneous stimulation methods (e.g., massage, pressure, or rubbing with soft cloth) to relieve the urge to scratch

- Keep room humidity at 30% to 40% and room temperature cool
- Cotton clothing and sheets should be washed in hypoallergenic soaps
- Distractions such as music, imagery, or relaxation may ease the itch sensation
- Medications may help relieve itch, depending on cause (antihistamines and corticosteroid for drug reaction; cholestyramine for biliary obstruction)

❏ *Photosensitivity*
  ☐ Manifestations
  - Exposed area becomes erythematous within a few hours; erythema gradually subsides
  - Rarely, photoallergy similar to contact dermatitis with immediate wheal-and-flare reactions or delayed reactions
  - With dacarbazine, pruritis and erythematous edematous eruptions of face, neck, and dorsal surfaces of both hands occur with sun exposure within 1 to 2 hours following drug administration
  ☐ Treatment
  - Obtain complete list of all medications patient has recently taken or is currently taking
  - Educate patients about dangers of exposure to UV radiation following treatment with radiation or certain chemotherapeutic agents

- Provide verbal and written instructions regarding ways to reduce risk

  Avoid tanning booths

  Limit exposure to sun

  Wear protective clothing and hats

  Use sunscreens properly

❏ *Vesicant chemotherapy extravasation*
  ☐ Prevented by
    - Professional training in chemotherapy drug administration
    - Having available guidelines for management
    - Following management guidelines in event of true or suspected extravasation
    - Completing documentation tool and establishing follow-up
  ☐ Manifestations
    - Bleb formation
    - Pain
    - Stinging or burning
    - Lack of blood return
    - Persistent complaints of pain or discomfort at site despite blood return
  ☐ Treatment
    - Stop drug administration
    - Disconnect chemotherapy drug infusion, connect syringe, and attempt to aspirate any blood or residual drug in tubing and at site
    - If you are unable to aspirate any blood, remove needle

- Apply sterile 2- × 2-inch gauze pad at site
- If antidote exists, prepare antidote and inject into preexisting syringe; if syringe has been removed, inject into site

  Nitrogen mustard: antidote is sodium thiosulfate

  Vinblastine: antidote is hyaluronidase

  Vincristine: antidote is hyaluronidase

- Remove needle
- Avoid application of direct manual pressure to site
- Photograph site
- Apply warm pack for 15 minutes 4 times daily for 24 hours if hyaluronidase has been used
- Apply cold pack for 15 minutes or more every 3 to 4 hours for 24 to 48 hours as tolerated for all other extravasations
- Notify physician that true or suspected extravasation has occurred
- Elevate extremity for 48 hours
- After 48 hours, instruct patient to use extremity to prevent contracture formation
- Arrange for return appointment once or twice weekly to monitor site
- Consult surgeon if pain persists beyond 7 to 10 days
- If extravasation has occurred from central line, stop infusion and notify physician

3. Malignant wounds

❏ *Manifestions*

- ☐ Excessive purulent drainage
- ☐ Odor
- ☐ Infection
- ☐ May progress to tissue ischemia and necrosis

❏ *Management*

- ☐ Surgery, radiation, chemotherapy, and hyperthermia
- ☐ *Debridement:* Necrotic tissue and eschar are removed to reduce infection and odor
- ☐ Topical or systemic antibiotics to control infection
- ☐ *Hemostasis:* Bleeding is most often result of trauma and can usually be prevented by proper wound care
- ☐ Odor management
  - ▪ Frequent cleaning
  - ▪ Topical chlorophyll-containing ointment and solutions
  - ▪ Charcoal-impregnated dressings
  - ▪ Room deodorizers
- ☐ Cleansing with solutions designed to minimize infection and odor
- ☐ Wound dressings
  - ▪ Maintain moist environment to prevent trauma from drying
  - ▪ Stimulate epithelial-cell migration and resurfacing

■ Hair

1. Assessment

❑ *For patient's risk of hair loss related to therapy*

❑ *For impact of hair loss on patient and significant others*

2. Prevention

❑ *Scalp hypothermia and scalp tourniquet cause vasoconstriction; neither method has proved particularly useful and they are not widely employed*

❑ *Hair preservation techniques are not recommended for patients with hematologic malignancies*

3. Nursing interventions

❑ *Inform patient of precise time of hair loss and how it will occur if possible*

❑ *Explain rationale for alopecia specific to therapy*
  □ Why hair falls out with specific therapy
  □ Variability of hair loss depending on therapy
  □ Possibility of hair regrowth—stress regrowth when appropriate
  □ Potential change in color and texture of new hair when regrowth occurs

❑ *Provide written literature*

❑ *Encourage patient to speak with others who have experienced and adjusted to hair loss*

❏ *Offer tips to minimize degree of alopecia*
  ☐ Shampoo gently 1 to 2 times/week with mild protein-based shampoo. Check with radiation therapist before washing hair if marks have been placed on scalp
  ☐ Rinse well with lukewarm water and gently pat dry with soft towel
  ☐ Use soft-bristled hairbrush or wide-toothed comb to reduce stress on hair shaft
  ☐ Use satin pillowcase to minimize rubbing friction on scalp hair while lying down
  ☐ Avoid use of hot rollers, hair dryers, curling irons, permanents, and hair dyes
  ☐ Avoid rollers in hair while sleeping, braids, ponytails, or cornrows
  ☐ Consider short haircut
  ☐ Utilize hair-preserving measures when appropriate

❏ *Provide information regarding wigs or hairpieces prior to hair loss*
  ☐ Types of wigs
  ☐ Cost, fit, and style
  ☐ Area retailers or available wig banks
  ☐ Reimbursement

❏ *Identify wig alternatives*
  ☐ Scarves, turbans, bandannas, sports caps, hats
  ☐ Use of wardrobe, makeup, and jewelry to highlight other features

❏ *Encourage use of eyebrow pencil, false eyelashes, wide-brimmed eyeglasses to minimize loss of eyebrows and eyelashes*

❏ *Inform patient of American Cancer Society's "Look Good . . . Feel Better Program"*

❏ *Instruct patient on ways to reduce trauma to remaining hair and skin of exposed scalp*

  ☐ Wash scalp gently with mild shampoo 1 to 2 times/week

  ☐ Use head covering to protect scalp from wind, cold, and sun

  ☐ Always apply sunscreen with SPF of 15 or more when sun exposure is expected

  ☐ While receiving radiation therapy, apply water-soluble, mild lubricant such as Natural Care Gel (Catalin Corp.), or Skin Balm (Carrington Laboratories) 2 to 3 times daily (do not apply 3 hours before receiving treatment)

  ☐ With chemotherapy cycles or after radiation treatments are completed, apply hydrophilic lubricant containing no perfume 2 to 3 times daily. Continue applying until hair regrowth begins

  ☐ Ensure wig lining is comfortable and nonirritating

❏ *Instruct patient on measures to protect eyes from injury (e.g., use of sunglasses, wide-brimmed hats, false eyelashes)*

❏ *Although controversial and limited in success, hair transplantation by punch or graft technique is only reported treatment for permanent radiation-induced alopecia*

■ **Nails**

1. **Inform patient of potential changes**
   ❑ *Decreased growth rates*
   ❑ *Development of ridges*

■ **Glands**

1. **Protect dry, irradiated skin as it is more susceptible to fissuring, infection, and necrosis from lack of lubrication by sweat and sebaceous glands**

Suggested Readings

1. Goodman M, Ladd LA, Purl S: Integumentary and mucous membrane alterations. In Groenwald SL, Frogge MH, Goodman M, Yarbro CH (eds.): *Cancer Nursing: Principles and Practice* (3rd ed.). Boston: Jones and Bartlett, 1993, pp. 734–799.

2. Perez CA, Brady LW: *Principles and Practice of Radiation Oncology* (2nd ed.). Philadelphia: Lippincott, 1992.

3. Dow KH, Hilderley LJ: *Nursing Care in Radiation Oncology*. Philadelphia: WB Saunders, 1992.

4. Eaglstein W, Rudolph R, Shannon ML: New directions in wound healing. *Wound Care Manual* 1:1–99, 1990.

5. Dorr RT: Antidotes to vesicant chemotherapy extravasation. *Blood Rev* 4:41–60, 1990.

▪ 22 ▪
Malignant Cerebral Edema

Overview

▪ Results from increase in fluid content of brain

▪ Metastasis to brain is prime source of cerebral edema

▪ Usually accompanies primary or metastatic brain tumors or carcinomatous meningitis

▪ Primary tumors that metastasize to brain most often are

1. Lung

2. Breast

3. Melanoma

4. Renal carcinoma

▪ Cerebral edema can result from

1. Direct injury to vascular endothelium

2. Dysplastic vascular structures within tumor

3. Biochemical alteration of capillary permeability

4. Unstable blood-brain barrier integrity

■ Tumors can continuously produce edema fluid

■ When cerebral edema exceeds compensatory limits of brain, herniation occurs

Approaches to Care

■ Assessment

1. Clinical manifestations
   ❏ *Headache*
   ❏ *Weakness*
   ❏ *Mental disturbance*
   ❏ *Seizure*
   ❏ *Gait disorder*
   ❏ *Visual disturbance*
   ❏ *Language disturbance*
   ❏ *Hemiparesis*
   ❏ *Impaired cognition*
   ❏ *Sensory loss (unilateral)*
   ❏ *Papilledema*
   ❏ *Ataxia*
   ❏ *Aphasia*

2. Diagnostic measures
   ❏ *Neurologic examination*

   ❏ *CT scan*

❑ *MRI—most definitive test*

❑ *Stereotactic needle biopsy may be required for tissue diagnosis*

■ **Interventions**

1. **Aggressive therapy to maintain optimal neurologic function**

2. **Radiation therapy is principal treatment**

   ❑ *Focused port*

   ❑ *Whole brain included in radiation field*

   ❑ *Treatment usually lasts 2 to 3 weeks*

   ❑ *Interstitial brachytherapy with seeds (iodine 120 or iridium) to boost field sometimes*

3. **Steroids to reduce edema**

   ❑ *Rapidly reduce rate of edema fluid formation*

   ❑ *Reduce intracranial pressure*

   ❑ *Increase cerebral blood flow*

   ❑ *Tapered once neurologic symptoms are controlled and reduced*

4. **Surgical decompression may be used for refractory situations**

   ❑ *Significant risks: infection, hemorrhage, operative mortality*

5. **Nursing management**

   ❑ *Assessment*

   ❑ *Side-effect management*

   ❑ *Safety and seizure precautions*

❏ *Prevention of complications of immobility*

❏ *Changes in vital signs are warning signs of intercranial hypertension*

❏ *Early detection of brain herniation*
   ☐ Decreased level of consciousness
   ☐ Change in pupil size
   ☐ Altered motor response

Suggested Readings

1. Maxwell MB: Malignant effusions and edema. In Groenwald SL, Frogge MH, Goodman M, Yarbro CH (eds.): *Cancer Nursing: Principles and Practice* (3rd ed.). Boston: Jones and Bartlett, 1993, pp. 690–693.

2. Weismann DE: Glucocorticoid treatment for brain metastases and epidural spinal cord compression: A review. *J Clin Oncol* 6:543–551, 1988.

3. Reulen HJ, Huber P, Ito U, et al: Peritumoral brain edema. In Long D, et al (eds.): *Advances in Neurology* (Vol 52.). New York: Raven Press, 1990.

4. Saba MT, Magolan JM: Understanding cerebral edema: Implications for oncology nurses. *Oncol Nurs Forum* 18:499–505, 1991.

■ 23 ■
Malignant Pericardial Effusion

Overview

■ Fluid accumulation in pericardial sac

■ Not often detected before death

■ Most patients are asymptomatic or have nonspecific symptoms

■ Only 8% to 20% develop metastasis to pericardium; of these, only one-third will develop symptoms of pericardial effusion

■ Types of tumors associated with pericardial effusion

1. Lung
2. Breast
3. Leukemia and lymphoma
4. Sarcoma
5. Melanoma

■ **Causes include**

1. **Pericardial metastasis**

2. **Direct invasion by adjacent tumor**

3. **Radiation-induced fibrotic obstruction**

■ **Effects are related to**

1. **Rate of fluid accumulation**

2. **Physical compliance of cavity**

3. **Cardiac efficacy**

4. **Interference with cardiac function by reducing volume of heart in diastole**

Approaches to Care

■ **Assessment**

1. **Clinical manifestations**

   ❏ *Tachycardia to offset stroke volume*

   ❏ *Systemic and pulmonary venous pressure increase to improve ventricular filling*

   ❏ *Increased blood pressure*

   ❏ *Dyspnea*

   ❏ *Cough*

   ❏ *Chest pain*

   ❏ *Orthopnea*

   ❏ *Weakness*

❏ *Dysphagia*

❏ *Syncope*

❏ *Palpitations*

❏ *Pleural effusion*

❏ *Jugular venous distention*

❏ *Hepatomegaly*

❏ *Peripheral edema*

❏ *Paradoxical pulse*

2. Diagnostic measures

❏ *Echocardiography, premature contractions, low QRS voltage, and nonspecific ST and T wave changes*

❏ *Pericardiocentesis for pericardial fluid; fluid usually has a bloody appearance*

❏ *Cytologic examination*

▥ Treatment

1. Dictated by degree of tamponade

2. If patient is asymptomatic, most clinicians wait and watch

3. If patient is symptomatic, treat to remove fluid and prevent its reaccumulation

4. To remove pericardial fluid, therapies are

❏ *Pericardiocentesis alone*
  ☐ Guided by echocardiography
  ☐ Needle is inserted into pericardial sac
  ☐ Fluid is aspirated

☐ Fluid will reaccumulate in short time

☐ Procedure is critical if tamponade is occurring

❏ *Subxiphoid pericardiotomy*

☐ Allows for longer period of drainage, examination of space

☐ Direct biopsy

5. **To obliterate pericardial space, therapies are**

❏ *Pericardiocentesis with sclerosing agent installation*

☐ Associated with significant toxicity

☐ Agents are tetracycline, 5-fluorouracil, radioactive gold or phosphorous, quinacrine, and thiotepa

☐ Fluid reaccumulates in 50% of cases

❏ *Surgery*

☐ Pleuropericardial window for effusions unresponsive to other treatments

☐ Pericardiectomy can also be done

❏ *Radiation*

☐ Lymphomas are extremely radiosensitive

☐ Effective in 50% of cases

☐ Breast and lung cancers may also respond

6. **Nursing measures**

❏ *Support patient and family through anxious period*

❏ *Maintain optimal cardiac output and function*

❏ *Prevent infection from invasive procedures*

❏ *Reduce patient's pain*

Suggested Readings

1. Maxwell MB. Malignant effusions and edema. In Groenwald SL, Frogge MH, Goodman M, Yarbro CH (eds.): *Cancer Nursing: Principles and Practice* (3rd ed.). Boston: Jones and Bartlett, 1993, pp. 684–687.

2. Hawkins JW. Vacek JL: What constitutes definitive therapy of malignant pericardial effusion? Medical vs surgical treatment. *Am Heart J* 118:428–432, 1989.

3. Joiner GA, Kolodychuk GR: Neoplastic cardiac tamponade. *Crit Care Nurs* 11:50–58, 1991.

▪ 24 ▪
Malignant Peritoneal Effusion

Overview

- Commonly referred to as *ascites*
- Occurs when volume of fluid that accumulates in peritoneal space exceeds capacity of lymphatic channels to drain
- Uncomfortable and most common with ovarian cancer
- Develops in over 60% of ovarian cancer patients
- Usually sign of advanced disease
- Tumors associated with peritoneal effusion are

1. Ovarian
2. Gastric
3. Endometrial
4. Pancreatic

5. Breast
6. Lymphoma
7. Colon
8. Mesothelioma

■ **Causes include**

1. Tumor seeding peritoneum

2. Excess intraperitoneal fluid production

3. Humoral factors produced by tumor cause increased capillary leakage of proteins and fluids into peritoneum

4. Hypoalbuminemia and low serum protein

Approaches to Care

■ **Assessment**

1. **Clinical manifestations**

   ❑ *Several liters of fluid can accumulate in peritoneal space*

   ❑ *Pressure and restrictiveness are hallmark symptoms*

   ❑ *Fullness*

   ❑ *Early satiety*

   ❑ *Indigestion*

   ❑ *Swollen ankles*

   ❑ *Fatigue*

   ❑ *Shortness of breath*

   ❑ *Constipation*

   ❑ *Reduced bladder capacity*

   ❑ *Weight gain*

- ❏ *Distended abdomen*
- ❏ *Fluid wave*
- ❏ *Shifting dullness*
- ❏ *Bulging flanks*
- ❏ *Everted umbilicus*

2. Diagnostic measures
- ❏ *Physical examination*
- ❏ *Paracentesis*
- ❏ *Fluid cytology*

■ Treatment

1. Only effective therapy is control of primary disease

2. If patient is asymptomatic, wait and see

3. If patient is symptomatic, initiate definitive therapy

4. Ascites fluid can be removed by

- ❏ *Paracentesis*
  - ☐ Fluid will reaccumulate rapidly
  - ☐ Risk that protein depletion and electrolyte abnormality will occur
  - ☐ Risk of infection

- ❏ *Obliteration of intraperitoneal space*
  - ☐ Instillation of chemotherapeutic agents; e.g., cisplatin
  - ☐ Administered intraperitoneally

- ☐ Peritoneovenous shunting
  - ■ Used to recirculate ascitic fluid to intravascular space
  - ■ Reserved for patients for whom other treatment options failed
  - ■ Complications
    Disseminated intravascular coagulation
    Infection
    Shunt malfunction

Suggested Readings

1. Maxwell MB. Malignant effusions and edema. In Groenwald SL, Frogge MH, Goodman M, Yarbro CH (eds.): *Cancer Nursing: Principles and Practice* (3rd ed.). Boston: Jones and Bartlett, 1993, pp. 687–690.

2. Ratliff CR, Hutchinson M, Conner C: Rapid paracentesis of large volumes of ascitic fluid. *Oncol Nurs Forum* 18:1461, 1991.

3. Hrozencik SP, Ness EA: Intraperitoneal chemotherapy via the Groshong catheter in the patient with gynecologic cancer. *Oncol Nurs Forum* 18:1245, 1991.

4. Kehoe C: Malignant ascites: Etiology, diagnosis, and treatment. *Oncol Nurs Forum* 18:523–530, 1991.

■ 25 ■
Malignant Pleural Effusion

Overview

■ Malignant pleural effusion occurs when malignant process prevents reabsorption and fluid accumulates in intrapleural space

■ May be initial symptom of cancer or may signal advanced disease

■ Typically recurs unless underlying disease is controlled or cured

■ Fifty percent of lung cancer patients develop effusion

■ Occurs most frequently with following tumors (in order of incidence):

1. Lung

2. Breast

3. Adenocarcinoma

4. Leukemia, lymphoma

5. Reproductive tract

6. Gastrointestinal tract

7. Primary unknown

■ Causes of malignant pleural effusion

1. Implantation of cancer cells on pleural surface

2. Tumor obstruction of lymphatic channels

3. Tumor obstruction of pulmonary veins leads to increased capillary hydrostatic pressure

4. Necrotic tumor cells shed into pleural space and increase osmotic pressure

5. Thoracic duct perforation

Approaches to Care

■ Assessment

1. Clinical manifestations
   - ❏ *Dyspnea*
   - ❏ *Orthopnea*
   - ❏ *Dry, nonproductive cough*
   - ❏ *Chest pain, heaviness*
   - ❏ *Labored breathing*
   - ❏ *Tachypnea*
   - ❏ *Dullness to percussion*
   - ❏ *Restricted chest wall*
   - ❏ *Impaired transmission of breath sounds*

2. Diagnostic measures
   - ❏ *Chest x-ray films*
   - ❏ *Pleural fluid cytology*

❏ *Thoracoscopy with direct pleural biopsy*

❏ *Bloody effusion is strongest indicator of malignancy*

◼ Interventions

1. **Definite treatment is based on tumor type and previous therapy**

   ❏ *If tumor causing effusion is responsive, systemic chemotherapy is initiated*

   ❏ *If tumor is questionably responsive, trial of systemic chemotherapy is initiated and thoracostomy tube is inserted to relieve symptoms*

   ❏ *If tumor is refractory to treatment, thoracostomy tube is inserted and pleurodesis is performed*

2. **Short-term relief of symptoms is accomplished by**

   ❏ *Thoracentesis*
   - ☐ Pleural fluid is removed by needle aspiration or via implanted port through chest wall
   - ☐ Complications include pneumothorax, pain, hypotension, or pulmonary edema
   - ☐ Effective for diagnosis, palliation, or relief of acute distress

   ❏ *Thoracostomy tube*
   - ☐ Inserted to remove fluid
   - ☐ Can be left in place to assess degree of fluid accumulation
   - ☐ Can be used to instill sclerosing agents

3. Sclerosing the pleural space

❏ *Is aggressive measure to prevent fluid reaccumulation*

❏ *Instillation of chemical agent causes visceral and parietal pleura to become permanently adhered together*

❏ *Sclerosing agents most commonly used are bleomycin and tetracycline*

❏ *Other agents include*
- ☐ Adriamycin
- ☐ Dactinomycin
- ☐ 5-Fluorouracil
- ☐ Nitrogen mustard
- ☐ Thiotepa
- ☐ Colloidal radioisotopes

4. Surgical methods

❏ *Used when above measures are unsuccessful*

❏ *Pleurectomy is effective in some cases*

❏ *Pleuroperitoneal shunt can also be inserted to divert pleural fluid into subcutaneous tissue via valved pump*

5. Radiation

❏ *Used if underlying tumor is responsive to radiotherapy*

❏ *Pulmonary fibrosis is potential complication*

Suggested Readings

1. Maxwell MB: Malignant effusions and edema. In Groenwald SL, Frogge MH, Goodman M, Yarbro CH (eds.): *Cancer Nursing: Principles and Practice* (3rd ed.). Boston: Jones and Bartlett, 1993, pp. 679–684.

2. Olopade OI, Ultmann JE: Malignant effusions. *CA* 41:166–179, 1991.

3. Moores DW: Malignant pleural effusion. *Semin Oncol* 18(suppl.):59–61, 1991.

4. Ruckdeschel JC: Management of malignant pleural effusion: An overview. *Semin Oncol* 15(3)(suppl.):24–28, 1988.

■ 26 ■
Mucous Membrane Alterations

Overview

■ Stomatitis

1. Risk factors

- ❏ *Dose-intensive chemotherapy*

- ❏ *Radiation therapy to head and neck region*

- ❏ *Higher doses of stomatotoxic drugs: 5-fluorouracil, methotrexate, bleomycin, doxorubicin, vinblastine, cytosine arabinoside, taxol*

- ❏ *Comcomitant administration of radiation and chemotherapy*

- ❏ *Liver or kidney dysfunction that may alter metabolism or elimination of stomatotoxic drug*

- ❏ *Higher doses of radiation given over shorter periods*

❏ *Poor nutritional status*

❏ *Tobacco and alcohol use*

2. **Risk of oral cavity infections after radiation or chemotherapy, or both, is directly related to degree and duration of granulocytopenia**

3. **Immunosuppression from treatment further increases susceptibility to oral infection**

■ **Xerostomia**

1. **Salivary glands highly sensitive to radiation**

2. **Decrease in quantity and quality of saliva**

■ **Taste changes**

1. **Chemotherapy and radiation cause direct injury to taste cells that results in taste changes**

2. **Radiation taste changes can be long-term, even permanent**

■ **Esophagitis**

1. **Both chemotherapy and radiation damage sensitive epithelial cells lining esophagus**

2. **Risk factors**

❏ *Stomatotoxic drugs: Dactinomycin, doxorubicin, 5-fluorouracil, methotrexate, hydroxyurea, procarbazine, vinblastine, taxol, and taxotere*

❏ *Concomitant chemotherapy and radiation to esophagus*

❑ *Alcohol consumption, tobacco use*

❑ *Ulcer disease*

■ Enteritis

1. **Three to five bowel movements daily or bowel movements of loose or watery consistency**

2. **Risk factors**

   ❑ *High-dose radiation to gastrointestinal (GI) tract*

   ❑ *Large volume field*

   ❑ *Concomitant chemotherapy and radiation therapy*

   ❑ *Chemotherapeutic agents most likely to cause diarrhea include*
   - ☐ 5-fluorouracil
   - ☐ Methotrexate
   - ☐ Cytosine arabinoside
   - ☐ Dactinomycin
   - ☐ Doxorubicin
   - ☐ Floxuridine

   ❑ *Poor nutrition, preexisting bowel disorders, diabetes, and hypertension may enhance enteritis*

3. **Other causes of diarrhea in cancer patient include**

   ❑ *Acute graft-versus-host disease*
   ❑ *Radiation*
   ❑ *Antibiotics*
   ❑ *Fecal impaction*
   ❑ *GI mucosal changes*

◼ Genitourinary mucositis

1. Cystitis and urethritis can occur in patients
   who have had radiation to prostate, cervix,
   and bladder

2. Vaginitis can occur in women who have
   radiation for gynecologic and colorectal
   malignancies

Approaches to Care

◼ Stomatitis

1. **Assessment**

   ❏ *Conduct dental evaluation and prophylactic
   care prior to treatment*

   ❏ *Care for periodontal disease prior to treatment
   with radiation or chemotherapy*

   ❏ *Daily fluoride treatments and good oral hygiene
   can reduce incidence of oral complications*

   ❏ *During treatment, assess oral cavity daily*

2. **Clinical manifestations**

   ❏ *Histologic changes within 5 to 7 days of
   exposure*

   ❏ *Inflammation and oral ulceration at 7 to 10
   days*

   ❏ *Resolution within 2 to 3 weeks*

   ❏ *If healing does not proceed, secondary
   infection leading to sepsis can occur*

   ❏ *Oral pain is major clinical problem*

3. Management

❏ *Treatment is palliative*

❏ *Depends on severity or grade of toxicity*

◻ *Grade 0:* potential stomatitis

▪ Encourage routine oral hygiene regimen after meals and at bedtime

Brush with soft toothbrush

Floss with unwaxed dental floss

Rinse with mouthwash of patient preference—avoid mouthwashes with high alcohol content

Remove, cleanse, and replace dental prostheses after oral care; store nightly in denture antiseptic solution

Apply lip lubricant

▪ Use oxidizing agent as needed

Three percent hydrogen peroxide and water (1:4 mixture)—swish, gargle, and expectorate

Sodium bicarbonate solution (e.g., 1 tsp in 8 oz water)—swish, gargle, and expectorate

Rinse with warm water or saline

Remove thick, tenacious mucus with swab as needed

▪ Use prophylactic chlorhexidine mouth rinse 15 ml—high-risk patients should swish, gargle, and expectorate every 8 hours

▪ Consult dentist

☐ *Grade 1:* erythema of oral mucosa, and
  Grade 2: isolated small ulcerations

  ▪ Assess oral cavity twice daily

  ▪ Follow oral hygiene regimen (see above)
    every 2 hours while awake and every 6
    hours during night

    *Use normal saline mouthwash if no crusts
      are present*

    *Alternate oxidizing agent with warm saline
      mouthwash if crusts are present*

    *Omit flossing if pain results or bleeding
      occurs with a low platelet count*

    *Remove, cleanse, and do not replace dental
      prostheses except for meals; store nightly
      in denture antiseptic solution*

  ▪ Culture suspicious oral lesions

  ▪ Apply topical anesthetics before meals and
    as needed for local pain control

  ▪ Use oral analgesics for systemic pain
    control

  ▪ Adapt diet to ensure maximum nutrition
    and fluid intake

    Encourage frequent small feedings

    Soft, bland foods

    Increase fluids to 3 liters/day

    Diet should be high in protein and calories

    Avoid irritants

    Consult dietitian as needed

☐ *Grade 3:* confluent ulcerations covering more
  than 25% of oral cavity or *Grade 4:*
  hemorrhagic ulceration

  ▪ Assess oral cavity every 8 hours

- Assess for evidence of infection; culture any suspicious lesion(s)

- Institute aggressive and timely antimicrobial therapy as ordered by physician

- Cleanse mouth every 2 hours while awake and every 4 hours at night

  Alternate warm saline mouthwash with antifungal or antibacterial oral suspension

  Use oxidizing agent for mucolytic area every 4 hours followed by saline rinse

- Gently brush teeth every 4 hours, avoiding trauma to gums; substitute soft foam toothettes if bleeding occurs or brushing is too painful

- Apply lip lubricant every 2 hours; if lips are bleeding or ulcerated, apply warm saline soaks every 4 hours for 20 minutes

- Remove and cleanse dental prostheses—do not replace; store in denture antiseptic solution

- Institute local pain control measures

- Use systemic analgesics as needed, especially after meals

- Provide adequate nutritional and fluid intake

  Liquid or pureed diet

  Intravenous fluids to prevent dehydration

  Enteral or total parenteral nutrition may be needed until healing occurs

- Frequency of oral care increases as severity of stomatitis increases

- Solutions commonly used to rinse oral
  cavity

  Normal saline

  Sodium bicarbonate

  Hydrogen peroxide

- Pain management includes local
  anesthetics (lidocaine, Cetacaine, or
  Hurricaine spray) and systemic analgesics
  depending on severity of oral discomfort

- Lip care includes moisture and lubrication

▇ Xerostomia

1. Manifestations

❑ *Mouth is dry, saliva becomes thick and ropey*

❑ *Nutrition, taste, and speech may be impaired*

❑ *Patient at risk for oral caries as well as
candidal infections*

2. Management

❑ *Assess oral cavity daily*

❑ *Instruct patient to*

  ☐ Increase fluids and eat soft or moistened food
    with milk or gravy

  ☐ Humidify air

  ☐ Avoid irritants such as tobacco, alcohol,
    carbonated beverages, and caffeine

  ☐ Take frequent sips of water to decrease oral
    irritation

  ☐ Use saliva substitutes

  ☐ Use sialagogues to stimulate secretion of saliva

▪ Taste changes

1. Manifestations

- ❑ *Patients complain of lowered threshold for bitter taste and increased threshold for sweet taste*

- ❑ *Metallic taste is commonly associated with cyclophosphamide*

2. Management: Instruct patient to

- ❑ *Engage in frequent and consistent oral hygiene*

- ❑ *Increase seasoning of food*

- ❑ *Use hard candy to mask taste associated with chemotherapy*

▪ Esophagitis

1. Manifestations

- ❑ *Dysphagia*

- ❑ *Odynophagia*

- ❑ *Epigastric pain may progress to ulceration, hemorrhage, and secondary infection*

- ❑ *Pain and difficulty swallowing can lead to dehydration and weight loss*

2. Management: Instruct patient to

- ❑ *Avoid hot, spicy, rough foods*

- ❑ *Eat foods that are soft and moist, like gravies*

- ❑ *Drink at least 8 glasses of fluid per day*

- ❑ *Humidify environment*

- ❑ *Avoid smoking or chewing any form of tobacco*

❑ *Take medicine prescribed for pain and discomfort*

❑ *Increase frequency of oral hygiene*

❑ *Tell physician about any dysphagia or pain, fever, or inability to drink fluids*

■ Enteritis

1. Manifestations

❑ *Chemotherapy-induced enteritis is manifested by diarrhea accompanied by abdominal cramping and rectal urgency*

❑ *Infection or antibiotic-associated colitis should be investigated and treated prior to antidiarrheal therapy that inhibits gut motility*

2. Management: Instruct patient to

❑ *Begin low-fat, low-fiber diet when symptoms occur*

❑ *Reduce or eliminate lactose from diet*

❑ *Use lactase enzyme caplets or lactose-free milk if helpful*

❑ *Avoid*
   ☐ Raw fruits and vegetables
   ☐ Cooked broccoli
   ☐ Butter
   ☐ Margarine
   ☐ Sauces
   ☐ Whole-grain breads
   ☐ Fatty foods
   ☐ Nuts
   ☐ Caffeine
   ☐ Alcohol

- [ ] Milk
- [ ] Milk products

❏ *Pharmacologic measures*
- [ ] Mild antidiarrheals such as Pepto-Bismol, Kaopectate, Lomotil, Imodium
- [ ] Opiates such as opium tincture, paregoric elixir, and codeine may decrease peristalsis
- [ ] Octreotide acetate (Sandostatin) given subcutaneously may control diarrhea by suppressing secretion of serotonin and gastroenteropancreatic peptides

■ Genitourinary mucositis

1. Urinary tract

❏ *Manifestations*
- [ ] Bladder irritation
- [ ] Dysuria
- [ ] Frequency and urgency
- [ ] Hemorrhagic cystitis from decreased capillary permeability and increased pressure of bloodflow

❏ *Treatment*
- [ ] Instruct patient to
  - Increase fluid intake
  - Use urinary anesthetics as needed
- [ ] Use antispasmodics

2. Vaginitis

❏ *Manifestations*
- [ ] Erythema
- [ ] Inflammation
- [ ] Atrophy

- ☐ Fibrosis
- ☐ Hypopigmentation
- ☐ Telangiectasia
- ☐ Inelasticity
- ☐ Ulceration
- ☐ Tissue necrosis, fistula formation, and hemorrhage can occur in patients who receive higher doses or radiation

❑ *Management: Instruct patient to*
- ☐ Dilate vagina with vaginal dilator or sexual intercourse
- ☐ Use good personal hygiene to minimize risk of secondary infection
- ☐ Report symptoms of vaginitis, such as vaginal discharge, itching, odor, pain, soreness, bleeding, or dyspareunia
- ☐ Use analgesics if needed to relieve severe discomfort or pain
- ☐ Use topical and systemic medications (miconazole nitrate or clotrimazole cream or suppositories)

Suggested Readings

1. Goodman M, Ladd LA, Purl S: Integumentary and mucous membrane alterations. In Groenwald SL, Frogge MH, Goodman M, Yarbro CH (eds.): *Cancer Nursing: Principles and Practice* (3rd ed.). Boston: Jones and Bartlett, 1993, pp. 734–799.

2. Perez CA, Brady LW: *Principles and Practice of Radiation Oncology* (2nd ed.). Philadelphia: Lippincott, 1992.

3. Dow KH, Hilderley LJ: *Nursing Care in Radiation Oncology.* Philadelphia: WB Saunders, 1992.

4. Beck SL: Prevention and managment of oral complications in the cancer patient. In Hubbard SM, Greene PE, Knopf MT (eds.): *Current Issues in Cancer Nursing Practice: Updates.* Philadelphia: Lippincott, 1992, pp. 1–11.

▪ 27 ▪
Nutritional Disturbances

Overview

■ Nutritional disturbances

1. Are a common consequence of cancer or its treatment

2. Predispose individuals to infection

3. Diminish patient's tolerance to therapy

4. Are important prognosticators of morbidity and survival

5. Are important issues in quality of life

■ Pathophysiology of malnutrition in cancer

1. Metabolic effects of tumor

   ❏ *Tumors produce peptides that cause cancer* cachexia

   ❏ *Carbohydrate, protein, and lipid metabolisms are altered*

❏ *Fluid and electrolyte abnormalities result from action of ectopic hormones*

❏ *Excessive energy requirements of tumors cause greater energy expenditures for individual*

❏ *Taste is altered*

❏ *Anorexia occurs in almost all cancer patients at some time during illness; this condition compounds weight loss and cachexia*

❏ *Immunosuppression occurs*

2. Mechanical effects of tumor

❏ *Expanding tumors cause local tissue damage with potential nutritional consequences such as*
   ☐ Infection
   ☐ Loss of appetite
   ☐ Nausea and vomiting
   ☐ Edema

3. Nutritional consequences of cancer treatment

❏ *Anorexia*

❏ *Constipation*

❏ *Diarrhea*

❏ *Fistulae*

❏ *Fluid and electrolyte imbalances*

❏ *Infection*

❏ *Malabsorption*
   ☐ Interruption of bowel structure
   ☐ Damage to absorptive surface of bowel
   ☐ Lack of substance necessary for absorption of nutrients

❑ *Mucositis*

❑ *Nausea and vomiting*

❑ *Taste changes*

Approaches to Care

▪ Nutritional assessment

1. Medical history

❑ *Duration and type of malignancy*

❑ *Frequency, type, and severity of complications (infections, draining lesions, etc.)*

❑ *Type and duration of therapy*

❑ *Specific chemotherapeutic agents used*

❑ *Radiation sites*

❑ *Antibiotics used*

❑ *Other drugs used*

❑ *Surgical procedures performed (site, type, and date)*

❑ *Side effects of therapy (diarrhea, anorexia, nausea and vomiting)*

❑ *Concomitant medical conditions (diabetes, heart disease, liver failure, kidney failure, infection)*

2. Physical examination

❑ *General appearance*

❑ *Condition of hair*

❑ *Condition of skin*

❑ *Condition of teeth*

❑ *Condition of mouth, gums, and throat*

❑ *Edema*

❑ *Performance status*

❑ *Identification of nutritionally related problems (fistula, pain, stomatitis, xerostomia, infection, constipation, diarrhea, nausea and vomiting, obstruction)*

3. Dietary history

❑ *Twenty-four-hour recall of foods eaten, including snacks*

❑ *Composition of food taken in 24 hours*

❑ *Time of day meals and snacks eaten*

❑ *Past or current diet modifications*

❑ *Self-feeding ability*

❑ *Special cancer diet*

❑ *Vitamins, minerals, or other supplements*

❑ *Modifications of diet or eating habits as result of treatment or illness*

❑ *Foods withheld or given on basis of personal or religious grounds*

❑ *Food preferences*

❑ *Food allergies or intolerances*

4. Socioeconomic history

❑ *Number of persons living in home*

❏ *Presence of kitchen facilities*
❏ *Income*
❏ *Food purchased by*
❏ *Food prepared by*
❏ *Amount spent on food per month*
❏ *Outside provision of meals*

5. Anthropometric data

❏ *Height*

❏ *Weight*

❏ *Actual weight as percentage of ideal*

❏ *Weight change as percentage of usual*

❏ *Triceps skinfold measurement (as indicator of subcutaneous body fat)*

❏ *Actual triceps skinfold as percentage of standard*

❏ *Midarm circumference (as index of protein status)*

❏ *Midarm muscle circumference*

❏ *Actual midarm muscle circumference as percentage of standard*

6. Biochemical data

❏ *Hematocrit*
❏ *Hemoglobin*
❏ *Serum albumin*
❏ *Serum transferrin*
❏ *Creatinine*
❏ *Creatinine height index*
❏ *Total lymphocyte count*
❏ *Delayed hypersensitivity response (skin testing)*

❏ *Nitrogen balance*
❏ *Blood urea nitrogen*
❏ *Sodium, potassium, carbon dioxide, chloride*
❏ *Glucose*

◼ Planning

1. **Identify goal of nutritional therapy**
2. **Establish individual's caloric requirements**
3. **Compose diet**

◼ Approaches to problems that interfere with normal nutrition

1. **Dysphagia: Encourage patient to**

   ❏ *Eat soft or liquid foods*

   ❏ *Blenderize solid foods*

   ❏ *Moisten foods with cream, gravies, or oils*

   ❏ *Eat bland foods that are smooth in texture and tepid to minimize pain*

2. **Nausea and vomiting: Encourage patient to**

   ❏ *Avoid acidic foods such as citrus juice and tomatoes*

   ❏ *Eat salty foods, or add salt to foods*

   ❏ *Avoid overly sweet, greasy, or high-fat foods*

   ❏ *Drink clear, cool beverages*

   ❏ *Eat dry foods such as toast or crackers, especially after getting up in morning*

   ❏ *Eat slowly and chew food thoroughly*

- ❏ *Eat small, frequent meals*

- ❏ *Eat frozen juice sticks or gelatin for fluid*

- ❏ *Rest with head elevated after eating*

- ❏ *Avoid rich, sweet foods*

- ❏ *Wear loose clothing*

- ❏ *Avoid favorite foods during chemotherapy to avoid developing aversion to them*

- ❏ *Take antinausea, antiemetic, tranquilizing medications as prescribed*

3. Early satiety: Encourage patient to

- ❏ *Eat five or six small meals per day*

- ❏ *Keep nutritious snacks available between meals*

- ❏ *Eat foods high in calories and low in fat*

- ❏ *Avoid greasy foods*

- ❏ *Chew foods slowly*

- ❏ *Avoid liquids with meals; take them half hour before or half hour after meals*

- ❏ *Drink nutritious liquids such as juice, milk, or milkshakes*

4. Pancreatic insufficiency: Encourage patient to

- ❏ *Take digestive enzymes as prescribed*

- ❏ *Follow a diet low in fat and high in calories and protein*

- ❏ *Take commercial food supplements as prescribed*

5. Anorexia: Encourage patient to

- ❏ *Eat small, frequent meals*
- ❏ *Make changes in diet or surroundings*
- ❏ *Try new recipes or foods, eat with friends, or go to favorite restaurant*
- ❏ *Stimulate appetite with light exercise*
- ❏ *Time meals to coincide with "best time" of day*
- ❏ *Eat nutritious, high-protein snacks*
- ❏ *Avoid "empty calorie" foods such as coffee or diet soda*
- ❏ *Take medications with high-calorie foods or nutritional supplements*
- ❏ *Add powdered milk to foods during cooking to increase protein content*
- ❏ *Drink small glass of wine or fruit juice before meals to stimulate appetite*
- ❏ *Avoid fatty foods*
- ❏ *Try foods served cold; they may be easier to tolerate*

6. Dumping syndrome: Encourage patient to

- ❏ *Eat foods low in concentrated carbohydrate, but high in protein*
- ❏ *Eat several small, dry meals during day*
- ❏ *Avoid liquids with meals; take them half hour before or half hour after meals*
- ❏ *Avoid sugar, candy, jam, jelly, honey, and desserts*

7. Constipation: Encourage patient to

- ❏ Drink at least 2 quarts of fluid daily
- ❏ Eat high-fiber foods
- ❏ Engage in light, regular exercise
- ❏ Take previously successful bowel stimulants

8. Diarrhea: Encourage patient to

- ❏ Drink plenty of fluids to avoid dehydration
- ❏ Avoid milk or milk products, unless they are treated with lactase enzyme
- ❏ Take electrolyte replacement fluids if diarrhea persists
- ❏ Avoid foods high in fiber
- ❏ Avoid high-fat, spicy, and gas-forming foods
- ❏ Eat foods rich in potassium

9. Dyspepsia: Encourage patient to

- ❏ Avoid fatty foods
- ❏ Avoid spicy foods
- ❏ Elevate upper trunk following meals
- ❏ Use antacids

10. Stomatitis: Encourage patient to

- ❏ Eat soft or liquid foods
- ❏ Avoid irritating foods that are rough or acidic
- ❏ Use warm saline irrigants to cleanse mouth
- ❏ Eat cold or frozen foods to numb pain
- ❏ Avoid extremely hot beverages

11. Taste changes: Encourage patient to

- ❏ Marinate red meat with sweet marinades or soy sauce

- ❏ *Substitute poultry, fish, eggs, or cheese for red meat*
- ❏ *Serve meats chilled rather than hot*
- ❏ *Use high-protein liquid supplements if meat is not tolerated*
- ❏ *Rinse mouth with carbonated water on a lemon wedge before meals to clear palate*
- ❏ *Eat mildly acidic foods such as lemonade, tea with lemon, pickled foods, and citrus fruits and juices to stimulate taste buds*
- ❏ *Try extra spices, onion, or garlic to improve flavor of food*
- ❏ *Keep experimenting; foods previously avoided may now be acceptable due to taste changes*

12. Xerostomia: Encourage patient to

- ❏ *Moisten foods with gravies or sauces*
- ❏ *Use artificial saliva as prescribed*
- ❏ *Use blender or food processor to make foods easier to eat*
- ❏ *Soak foods in coffee, tea, milk, cocoa, or warm beverages*
- ❏ *Avoid dry foods such as crackers or toast*
- ❏ *Swallow liquid with each bite of food*
- ❏ *Use humidifier or steam kettle in room where food is eaten*

13. **General: Encourage patient to**

   ❏ *Drink plenty of fluids*

   ❏ *Make mealtime pleasant with different surroundings and pleasant company*

   ❏ *Serve food attractively; use garnishes*

   ❏ *Experiment with recipes, flavoring, spices*

   ❏ *Avoid empty-calorie foods such as soda*

   ❏ *Eat high-calorie foods*

   ❏ *Take advantage of best time of day for eating*

   ❏ *Eat early in day if energy levels are higher then*

   ❏ *Keep nutritious snacks handy to increase nutrient intake*

■ Administration of nutritional therapy

1. **Oral feeding**

   ❏ *Regular diet is preferred if individual is able to consume adequate quantity of foods orally*

   ❏ *For those unable to eat adequate amounts, supplemental calories, protein, vitamins, and minerals may be indicated*

   ❏ *Liquid nutritional formulas may be used*

2. **Enteral (tube) feeding**

   ❏ *Indicated if oral intake cannot prevent weight loss, or if person's physical condition prevents oral intake*

   ❏ *Requires functioning gastrointestinal (GI) tract*

❏ *For tumors of head and neck, lung, or upper GI tract, feeding directly into small intestine may be indicated*

❏ *May be administered by nasogastric or nasointestinal means*

❏ *For more permanent feeding, surgically placed esophagostomy, gastrostomy, or jejunostomy tube may be indicated*

❏ *Formulas may be prepared from regular food, or may be commercially prepared*

❏ *Side effects tend to lessen over time, making enteral feeding appropriate for long-term use*
  □ Diarrhea
    - Attributed to formula-related factors including lactose content, bacterial contamination, and osmolality
    - If it does not resolve within 2 to 3 days, medical work-up may be indicated
    - Antidiarrheal medication may be prescribed
  □ Fluid and electrolyte disturbances may occur
    - Monitor fluid status daily
  □ Hyperglycemia may occur during initial stages of feeding and continue in individuals with diabetes
    - Monitor blood and urine glucose levels

3. Total parenteral nutrition (TPN)

❏ *Intravenous infusion of concentrated mixture of amino acids, glucose, fluid, vitamins, minerals, electrolytes, and trace elements into central vein, usually superior vena cava*

- ❏ *Indicated when enteral feedings are impossible due to nonfunctioning GI tract*

- ❏ *Allows bowel of individual on cancer therapy to rest, thereby allowing individual to complete course of therapy*

- ❏ *Complications*
  - ☐ Infection
    - ▪ From contamination of TPN solution, insertion site, or equipment
    - ▪ Offending organisms are usually skin microorganisms such as bacteria *Staphylococcus, Klebsiella,* and *Corynebacterium,* and fungi *Candida*
    - ▪ Early detection is an important nursing responsibility
    - ▪ First sign may be sudden glycosuria (or hyperglycemia) in previously stable individual
    - ▪ Clinical signs of sepsis include fever, hypotension, tachycardia, and tachypnea
    - ▪ If there is temperature spike, peripheral blood and blood drawn from catheter are cultured for bacteria and fungi
    - ▪ If culture is positive, catheter is assumed to be source of infection and is removed
    - ▪ New catheter not inserted until all blood cultures are negative
    - ▪ Bacterial sepsis treated with antibiotics
    - ▪ Fungal sepsis treated with fungicidal agent
  - ☐ Mechanical complications
    - ▪ Improper functioning of central line due to *Blockage of line from catheter crimping*

Thrombosis

Malfunction of infusion pump

Failure of infusion set

- Can be minimized if personnel are knowledgeable and skilled and if there is standardized protocol for care of TPN equipment

☐ Thrombosis of central vein

- Is a rare, but serious complication

- Requires prompt removal of catheter and administration of sodium heparin

- Signs include erythema, edema of catheter insertion site, pain along course of vein, fever, tachycardia, tachypnea, malaise, and ipsilateral swelling of arm, neck, or face

☐ Air embolism

- Is rare, but potentially fatal

- Is prevented by clamping tubing securely to prevent air from entering system

- Inspect infusion system regularly for leaks or cracks

- Signs of sudden vascular collapse are

Chest pain

Apprehension

Tachycardia

Hypotension

Cyanosis, progressing to seizures

Loss of consciousness

Cardiac arrest

- Immediate emergency nursing action is to position person on his or her left side with head down to allow air to dissipate gradually through pulmonary artery. Action may take several minutes, but eliminates vascular obstruction

☐ Metabolic complications

- Most common is *hyperglycemia,* which occurs in 15% of all individuals receiving TPN therapy. Results when

  Infusion is too rapid

  Insulin response is inadequate

  There are increased insulin demands on individual

  > Monitored with fractional urine tests or finger sticks for blood glucose every 6 hours

  > Symptoms include dry mouth, flushed skin, thirst, malaise, polyuria, nausea, or vomiting

  > Treated by addition of insulin to each TPN solution

- *Hypoglycemia* occurs when too much insulin is administered or when TPN infusion is interrupted or discontinued shortly after insulin is given

  Symptoms include headache, drowsiness, dizziness, tachycardia, and tremor

  Corrected when TPN infusion is balanced against insulin administration

- Essential fatty acid deficiency occurs as result of prolonged reduction of fat intake

Symptoms are

Scaling of skin over lower calf and dorsum of foot

Alopecia

Delayed wound healing

Increased capillary fragility

Thrombocytopenia

Deficiency is treated by administering lipid emulsion to individuals who receive TPN for longer than 14 days without dietary fat intake

Prevents essential fatty acid deficiency

Provides concentrated energy source

Is isotonic and therefore does not damage endothelium

Does not require insulin

Guidelines for lipid emulsion infusion

Do not use emulsion if color or texture is inconsistent

Do not shake container excessively

Nothing can be added to lipid infusion

Infuse in same line as TPN solution using Y-connector located near infusion site

Lipid infusion should be hung higher than TPN or it will run up TPN line

Do not use filter

Initial maximum rate of infusion is 1 cc/min for first 30 minutes. If there are no untoward reactions, increase to 500 cc over 4 to 12 hours

Observe for allergic reactions, dyspnea, cyanosis, nausea, vomiting, headache, flushing, fever, chills, pain in chest or back, irritation at infusion site, and diaphoresis; if any reactions occur, discontinue infusion

Discard remaining solution—do not store for later use

Suggested Readings

1. Skipper A, Szeluga DJ, Groenwald SL: Nutritional disturbances. In Groenwald SL, Frogge MH, Goodman M, Yarbro CH (eds.): *Cancer Nursing: Principles and Practice* (3rd ed.). Boston: Jones and Bartlett, 1993, pp. 620–643.

2. Lipman TO: Clinical trials of nutritional support in cancer: Parenteral and enteral therapy. *Heme/Oncol Clin North Am* 5:125–145, 1991.

3. Ropka M: Nutrition. In Gross J, Johnson BL (eds.): *Handbook of Oncology Nursing* (2nd ed.). Boston: Jones and Bartlett, 1994, pp. 329–372.

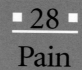

■ 28 ■
Pain

Overview

■ Pain is an unpleasant sensory and emotional experience associated with tissue damage

■ Chronic pain and acute pain are different

■ There are three types of pain in patients with cancer, each with a different etiology

1. **Tumor-related pain caused by**
   - ❑ *Infiltration of bone*
   - ❑ *Infiltration of nerves*
   - ❑ *Infiltration of intestinal tract and viscera*

2. **Treatment-related pain caused by**
   - ❑ *Diagnostic procedures*
   - ❑ *Surgery*
   - ❑ *Radiotherapy*
   - ❑ *Chemotherapy*
   - ❑ *Complications*

3. **Pain unrelated to either tumor or treatment**

◼ **Pain is most prevalent in patients with**

1. Advanced disease
2. Lung cancer
3. Breast cancer
4. Pancreatic cancer
5. Primary bone cancer

◼ **Obstacles to successful pain management include**

1. Lack of understanding about pain
2. Expectation that pain should be present
3. Relief of pain not viewed as goal of treatment
4. Inadequate or nonexistent assessment
5. Undertreatment with analgesics
6. Inadequate knowledge of drugs or other interventions
7. Fears of addiction, sedation, respiratory depression
8. Legal impediments

Approaches to Care

◼ **Assessment**

1. *Physiologic dimension*
   ❑ *Onset*

❏ *Duration*
  ☐ Acute pain: Self-limiting
  ☐ Chronic pain: Lasts 3 months or longer

❏ *Pattern*
  ☐ Brief or transient
  ☐ Periodic or intermittent
  ☐ Continuous or constant

2. *Sensory dimension*

❏ *Location of pain*

❏ *Intensity (e.g., mild, moderate, severe) of pain*

❏ *Quality (e.g., burning, stabbing, throbbing) of pain*

3. *Affective dimension*

❏ *Depression*   ❏ *Mental state*
❏ *Anxiety*

4. *Cognitive dimension*

❏ *Meaning of pain*
❏ *Coping strategies*
❏ *Knowledge, attitudes, beliefs*
❏ *Influencing factors (positive and negative)*

5. *Behavioral dimension*

❏ *Level of activity*
❏ *Use of medications*
❏ *Communication with others*
❏ *Sleep and rest patterns*
❏ *Behaviors to control pain*

6. *Sociocultural dimension*

❏ *Ethnocultural background*
❏ *Family and social life*

❑ *Work and home responsibilities*
❑ *Environment*
❑ *Familial attitudes, beliefs, and behaviors*
❑ *Personal attitudes, beliefs, and behaviors*

7. **The Oncology Nursing Society has described nurse's role as**

❑ *Describing pain*

❑ *Identifying aggravating and relieving factors*

❑ *Determining meaning of pain and its cause*

❑ *Determining individual's definition of pain relief*

❑ *Deriving nursing diagnoses*

❑ *Assisting in selection of interventions*

❑ *Evaluating efficacy of interventions*

8. **Standardized pain assessment tools and documentation procedures facilitate management of pain**

■ **Interventions**

1. **Treat underlying pathology by**

❑ *Chemotherapeutic agents to palliate symptoms*

❑ *Hormonal therapy to provide relief of painful bone metastases from breast and prostate cancers*

❑ *Radiotherapy to provide fast pain relief in patients with*
☐ Bone, brain, and hepatic metastases
☐ Epidural cord compression
☐ Nerve root infiltration

❑ *Surgery to*
  ☐ Resolve oncologic emergencies
  ☐ Reduce tumor burden
  ☐ Provide direct access to tumor (e.g., implants of infusion pumps or radiation seeds)

2. Pharmacologic therapy

❑ *Nonopioids*

  ☐ *Nonsteroidal anti-inflammatory drugs* (NSAIDs) used alone or with an opioid for
    ▪ Mild to moderate pain
    ▪ Metastatic bone pain
    ▪ Pain from compression of tendons, muscles, pleura, and peritoneum
    ▪ Visceral pain

  ☐ Commonly used nonopioids are
    ▪ Acetaminophen
    ▪ Acetylsalicylic acid
    ▪ Choline magnesium trisalicylate
    ▪ Diclofenac
    ▪ Diflunisal
    ▪ Ibuprofen
    ▪ Indomethacin
    ▪ Ketorolac
    ▪ Naproxen

  ☐ Major toxicities of NSAIDs are
    ▪ Gastrointestinal disorders: Nausea, vomiting, epigastric pain, ulcers, bleeding, diarrhea, constipation
    ▪ Renal dysfunction
    ▪ Sodium and water retention
    ▪ Skin rashes
    ▪ Headaches

❏ *Opioids*
- ❏ *Opioid agonists* are very useful for cancer pain and include
  - Codeine
  - Fentanyl
  - Hydromorphone
  - Methadone
  - Morphine
- ❏ *Morphine* is most frequently used opioid for moderate to severe pain and advantages include
  - Long-acting form with 8 to 12 hour dosing schedules
  - Flexibility in dosing with 15-, 30-, 60-, and 100-mg tablet sizes
  - Oral, parenteral, rectal, and intraspinal preparations
- ❏ Addiction is highly unlikely
- ❏ Most common side effects
  - Sedation
  - Respiratory depression (treat with naloxone)
  - Nausea and vomiting
  - Constipation

❏ *Adjuvant analgesics*
- ❏ *Antidepressants* are used for neuropathic pain (e.g., continuous burning) due to tumor infiltration of nerves. Agents include
  - Amitriptyline
  - Nortriptyline
  - Imipramine
  - Desipramine
  - Doxepin
  - Trazodone
  - Maprotiline

  ☐ *Anticonvulsants* are used for lancinating and
   stabbing-like neuropathic pain

    ■ Phenytoin   ■ Clonazepam
    ■ Carbamazepine ■ Valproic acid

  ☐ *Psychostimulants* counteract sedation of
   opioid analgesics

    ■ Amphetamines
    ■ Methylphenidate

3. Routes of opioid administration

 ❏ *Oral route*

  ☐ Convenient and safe
  ☐ Inexpensive
  ☐ Should be used as long as possible

 ❏ *Parenteral* (intramuscular, subcutaneous,
  intravenous) route

  ☐ Occasional intramuscular or subcutaneous
   injection if no peripheral or central venous
   access

  ☐ Consider continuous infusion if analgesic
   needed every 2 hours or less

  ☐ Continuous intravenous infusions provide
   steady blood levels of opioid

  ☐ Morphine and hydromorphone most common
   for continuous subcutaneous infusions

 ❏ *Transdermal route*

  ☐ Fentanyl only opioid available via this route

 ❏ *Rectal route*

 ❏ *Intraspinal route*

  ☐ Criteria for intraspinal opioids include

    ■ Unacceptable toxicities from systemic opioids

    ■ Neuroablative or anesthetic procedures
     unsuccessful or not indicated

- Good home and family support
- Life expectancy greater than 3 months

4. Patient-controlled analgesia (PCA)

❏ *Allows patient to self-administer analgesics from special infusion pump*

❏ *Used with intravenous, subcutaneous, and epidural route*

❏ *Avoids highs and lows of (PRN) administration*

❏ *Used by bolus dosing or bolus with continuous infusion*

❏ *Appropriate use for PCA*
  - ☐ When patient wants self-control
  - ☐ When oral route not available
  - ☐ For breakthrough pain

5. Anesthetic and nerve-block procedures

❏ *Prevent generation and conduction of nerve impulses*

❏ *Used for intractable pain*

6. Nonpharmacologic interventions

❏ *Do not affect pathology or alter sensation or perception of pain*

❏ *Practical components of nursing practice*

❏ *Selected interventions*
  - ☐ Counterirritant cutaneous stimulation
    - Mentholated ointments
    - Heat
    - Cold

- Massage
- Transcutaneous electrical nerve stimulation
☐ Immobilization and mobilization
☐ Distraction
  - Conversation
  - Visualization and imagery
  - Breathing exercises
  - Counting, reading, watching television
  - Speaking to others
☐ Relaxation and guided imagery
☐ Music therapy
☐ Laughter therapy
☐ Biofeedback
☐ Hypnosis

❏ *These techniques are used in conjunction with pharmacologic interventions and require careful assessment and evaluation*

Suggested Readings

1. McGuire DB, Sheidler VR: Pain. In Groenwald SL, Frogge MH, Goodman M, Yarbro CH (eds.): *Cancer Nursing: Principles and Practice.* Boston: Jones and Bartlett, 1993, pp. 499–556.

2. McCaffery M, Beebe a (eds.): *Pain: Clinical Manual for Nursing Practice.* St. Louis: CV Mosby, 1989.

3. Spross JA, McGuire DB, Schmidt R: Oncology Nursing Society position paper on cancer pain. *Oncol Nurs Forum* 17:595–614, 751–760, 825, 944–955, 1990.

■ 29 ■
Septic Shock

Overview

■ Results from *septicemia,* a systemic blood
infection

■ Characterized by

1. Hemodynamic instability

2. Coagulopathy

3. Altered metabolism

■ Incidence is increasing due to numerous
invasive procedures

■ Mortality rate is 75% for cancer patients who
develop septic shock

■ Risk factors include

1. Local effects of tumor growth

2. Immunologic effects of cancer or treatment

3. Granulocyte count less than $100/mm^3$

4. Iatrogenic factors

5. Nosocomial sources

6. Invasive procedures

Approaches to Care

▇ Assessment

1. Clinical manifestations

- ❏ *Early signs*
  - □ Tachycardia
  - □ Fever or hypothermia
  - □ Rigors
  - □ Hypertension

- ❏ *Late signs*
  - □ Bilateral rales
  - □ Oliguria
  - □ Evidence of inadequate tissue perfusion
  - □ Cyanosis, hypotension, mental changes
  - □ Adult respiratory distress syndrome

2. Diagnostic measures

- ❏ *Early identification is critical to prevent death*
- ❏ *Blood cultures to identify microorganisms*
- ❏ *Chest x-ray films*

▇ Treatment

1. Initiate empiric broad-spectrum antibiotic therapy immediately

2. Initial treatment usually includes aminoglycoside, penicillin, and cephalosporin

3. If *Staphylococcus epidermidis* is suspected, add vancomycin

4. If shock develops during prolonged antibiotic therapy, suspect fungal source and treat with amphotericin B

5. In 30% of cancer patients, infecting organism cannot be identified

6. Monitor vital signs, central venous or pulmonary artery pressure, and urine output

7. Vigorous fluid replacement expands volume

8. Fresh-frozen plasma increases mean arterial pressure

9. Give vasopressors if patient is unresponsive to fluid therapy

10. Corticosteroid therapy produces anti-inflammatory response

11. Give oxygen and monitor blood gases

12. Metabolic acidosis is possible

13. Mechanical ventilation may be needed

14. Effective therapy is measured by stable vital signs, adequate pressures, and urine output

15. Educate patient regarding preventive measures

Suggested Readings

1. Dietz KA, Flaherty AM: Oncologic emergencies. In Groenwald SL, Frogge MH, Goodman M, Yarbro CH (eds.): *Cancer Nursing: Principles and Practice* (3rd ed.). Boston: Jones and Bartlett, 1993, pp. 801–805.

2. Parrillo JE: Management of septic shock: Present and future. *Ann Intern Med* 115:491–493, 1991.

3. Truett L: The septic syndrome: An oncologic treatment challenge. *Cancer Nurs* 14:175–180, 1991.

4. Bone RC: a critical evaluation of new agents for the treatment of sepsis. *JAMA* 266:1686–1691, 1991.

Spinal Cord Compression

Overview

■ Occurs when tumor encroaches on spinal cord or cauda equina

■ Neurologic emergency requiring prompt diagnosis and treatment to preserve person's neurologic function

■ Can cause partial or complete paralysis if not recognized or treated early

■ Is classified according to location of tumor that is causing compression as intramedullary, intradural, extravertebral, or extradural

■ Site of compression is related to primary cancer

1. Cervical compression—breast

2. Thoracic compression—lung, breast, prostate

3. Lumbosacral—gastrointestinal (GI) cancers

■ Compression of spinal cord occurs either by direct extension of tumor into epidural space or by vertebral collapse and displacement of bony elements

■ About 5% of cancer patients develop spinal cord compression (SCC)

■ Over 95% of SCC cases are due to tumor that has metastasized to vertebral column

■ Risk factors

1. Tumors that metastasize to bone

2. Primary cancers are

- ❏ *Breast*
- ❏ *Lung*
- ❏ *Prostate*
- ❏ *GI cancer*
- ❏ *Unknown primary*
- ❏ *Sarcoma*
- ❏ *Neuroblastoma*
- ❏ *Thyroid*

Approaches to Care

■ Assessment

1. Clinical manifestations

- ❏ *Over 95% of SCC patients present with pain*
- ❏ *Pain is either radicular or localized*
- ❏ *Pain with or without neurologic symptoms can indicate degree of blockage of spinal cord*

❏ *Thoracic SCC is described as constrictive band around waist*

❏ *Pain is usually within one or two vertebrae of compression*

❏ *Radicular pain can follow dermatome of involved nerve root*

❏ *Motor weakness occurs in about 75% of patients and is rarely presenting symptom; usually described as heaviness or stiffness*

❏ *Sensory loss begins with numbness and paresthesia, but can progress to loss of light touch, pain, then thermal sensation*

❏ *Loss of proprioception, deep pressure, or position represents more severe cord compression*

❏ *Autonomic dysfunction includes bladder and bowel disturbances. Loss of sphincter control is most common*

2. Diagnostic measures

❏ *Pain can be elicited by percussion of vertebrae near SCC, or by either straight leg raising or neck flexion*

❏ *Pain is aggravated by coughing, sneezing, or Valsalva's maneuver*

❏ *Pain is not relieved by lying down*

❏ *Distinguishing pain as being due to SCC or metastases can be difficult*

❏ *Hallmark of SCC pain is pain that changes location, intensity, or nature*

❏ *Single most important prognostic indicator with SCC is neurologic status before initiation of therapy: the less extensive injury to cord, greater potential for recovery*

❏ *Assessment parameters include pain, sensory changes, muscle weakness, hyperreflexia, urinary changes, and bowel changes*

❏ *Spine film*

❏ *MRI is most definitive tool*

❏ *Myelography and computed tomographic scan are also used*

■ Treatment

1. Timely treatment is as important as rapid diagnosis

❏ *If treated early, neurologic deficits are rare*

❏ *Effective treatment is directly related to prolonged survival and quality of life*

2. Controversy exists regarding initial treatment of choice

❏ *Radiation therapy*
❏ *Surgical decompression*
❏ *Combined approach of surgery and radiation*

3. Radiation therapy

❏ *Most often used*

❏ *Total dose of 3000 to 4000 cGy is given to port that includes one or two vertebrae above and below compression*

❑ *Side effects are minimal unless patient has less than optimal bone marrow function, which may be suppressed further*

4. **Surgical decompression with laminectomy or vertebral body resection**

❑ *Used for prompt relief*

❑ *Used as first line of therapy if patient is neurologically unstable, tumor is radioresistant or previously irradiated, or spine is unstable*

❑ *Primary goal is decompression by providing alternate space for tumor and for spine stabilization*

5. **Surgery followed by radiation therapy appears to offer no greater advantage than radiotherapy alone**

6. **Steroids are included in any management approach**

❑ *Often given before definitive diagnosis is made*
❑ *Aid in reducing inflammation and edema*
❑ *Can have oncolytic effect*

7. **Pain management is achieved with pharmacologic and nonpharmacologic measures described in Chapter 28**

8. **Nursing measures**

❑ *Pain control*

❑ *Protection of patient from sensory, motor, or neurologic injury*

❏ *Rehabilitation*
  ☐ Depending on pretreatment status of patient, rehabilitation approaches vary
  ☐ If pretreatment neurologic status is poor, patient will not likely regain function
  ☐ Extensive rehabilitation can aid in maximizing recovery or providing adaptive measures

Suggested Readings

1. Dietz KA, Flaherty AM: Oncologic emergencies. In Groenwald SL, Frogge MH, Goodman M, Yarbro CH (eds.): *Cancer Nursing: Principles and Practice* (3rd ed.). Boston: Jones and Bartlett, 1993, pp. 829–836.

2. Siegal TA, Siegal TZ: Current considerations in the management of neoplastic spinal cord compression. *Spine* 14(2):223–228, 1989.

3. Glover D, Glick JH: Oncologic emergencies: Spinal cord compression. In Holleb AI, Fink DJ, Murphy GP (eds.): *American Cancer Society Textbook of Clinical Oncology*. Atlanta: American Cancer Society, 1991, pp. 513–533.

4. Dyck S: Surgical instrumentation as a palliative treatment for spinal cord compression. *Oncol Nurs Forum* 18(3):515–521, 1991.

■ 31 ■
Superior Vena Cava Syndrome

Overview

■ Obstruction of superior vena cava is usually due to

1. External compression by tumor or lymph nodes

2. Direct invasion of vessel wall by tumor

3. Thrombosis of vessel

■ Development of superior vena cava syndrome (SVCS) depends on

1. Degree and location of obstruction

2. Aggressiveness of tumor

3. Competency of collateral circulation

■ If untreated, SVCS can lead to

1. Thrombosis

2. Cerebral edema

3. **Pulmonary complications**

4. **Death**

◾ **SVCS may be presenting sign of malignancy**

◾ **Occurs in 3% to 4% of oncology patients, yet 97% of SVCS cases are due to cancer**

◾ **Risk factors**

1. **Lung cancer and lymphoma**

2. **Thrombus formation around central venous catheter**

3. **Radiation-induced fibrosis of vessel**

Approaches to Care

◾ **Assessment**

1. **Clinical manifestations**

❏ *Elevated venous pressure and congestion result in signs and symptoms that are hallmarks of this syndrome*

❏ *Severity of symptoms is related to rapidity of onset and adequacy of collateral circulation to reduce congestion*

❏ *Early signs and symptoms*
  ☐ Facial, trunk, and upper extremity edema
  ☐ Pronounced venous pattern on trunk
  ☐ Neck vein distention
  ☐ Cough

❏ *Late signs*
  □ Hoarseness
  □ Stridor
  □ Engorged conjunctiva
  □ Headache
  □ Dizziness
  □ Visual disturbances
  □ Changes in mental status
  □ Acute respiratory distress

2. Diagnostic measures

❏ *Chest x-ray film may reveal mediastinal mass or adenopathy*

❏ *Histopathologic diagnosis via biopsy or cytology if condition is not threatening*

■ Treatment

1. Immediate intervention to prevent respiratory arrest includes

❏ *High doses of fractionated radiation of mediastinum (300–400 cGy/dy)*

❏ *Doses may be tapered, but achieve cumulative 3000 to 3500-cGy dose*

2. For nonthreatening SVCS

❏ *Tissue diagnosis first*

❏ *Subsequent appropriate cancer therapy (e.g., small-cell lung cancer is chemosensitive and thus treated; if unresponsive, then radiation is given)*

3. Steroids are sometimes given to further reduce edema

4. Anticoagulants can prevent thrombosis secondary to decreased blood flow through vessel

5. Antifibrinolytics are sometimes given to reduce intramural thrombi

6. Catheter-induced SVCS is treated with fibrinolytic agents (streptokinase, urokinase, tissue plasminogen activator)

7. Surgical procedures, bypass graft, and stent placement are reserved for person with good prognosis for whom other options have been exhausted

8. Maintain adequate cardiopulmonary status

9. Monitor progression of SVCS

10. Reduce patient's anxiety

11. Avoid invasive or constrictive procedures of upper extremities
   ❏ Take blood pressure measurements on thigh
   ❏ Perform venipuncture on lower extremities

12. Administration of vesicant or irritant chemotherapy agents is controversial because lower extremities are used. Surgical cannulation of femoral vein is safest route if administration is necessary

13. Provide fluid therapy and diuresis therapy to avoid overload and further venous congestion

14. Position patient with head of bed elevated to help maximize breathing and allay anxiety

15. Provide calm environment with visible support, reinforcement of temporary nature of patient's physical appearance, and clear understanding of treatment plan

16. Resolution of syndrome usually occurs within 24 to 72 hours after therapy is initiated. If syndrome does not respond, thrombus formation is suspected and surgical intervention may be needed

17. Routine follow-up care is usually all that is needed once SVCS is resolved with effective therapy

Suggested Readings

1. Dietz KA, Flaherty AM: Oncologic emergencies. In Groenwald SL, Frogge MH, Goodman M, Yarbro CH (eds.): *Cancer Nursing: Principles and Practice* (3rd ed.). Boston: Jones and Bartlett, 1993, pp. 810–813.

2. Schaefer SL: Oncologic complications: Superior vena cava syndrome. In Otto SE (ed.): *Oncology Nursing*. St. Louis: Mosby Year Book, 1991, pp. 468–526.

3. Yahalom J: Oncologic emergencies: Superior vena cava syndrome. In DeVita VT, Hellman S, Rosenberg SA (eds.): *Cancer: Principles and Practice of Oncology* (3rd ed.). Philadelphia: Lippincott, 1989, pp. 1971–1977.

4. Greenberg S, Kosinski R, Daniels J: Treatment of SVC thrombosis with rTPA. *Chest* 99(5):1298–1301, 1991.

▪ 32 ▪
Syndrome of Inappropriate Antidiuretic Hormone

Overview

■ Paraneoplastic syndrome resulting from excessive amounts of antidiuretic hormone (ADH), which exerts significant effect on kidneys and results in water intoxication

■ Excess ADH can result from

1. Ectopic production

2. Abnormal stimulation of hypothalamus-pituitary network

3. ADH effects on kidney that are mimicked or enhanced

■ Results of water intoxication

1. Drop in plasma osmolality

2. Dilutional hyponatremia

3. Increased urinary excretion of sodium

4. Further hyponatremia

■ About 1% to 2% of cancer patients develop syndrome of inappropriate antidiuretic hormone (SIADH)

■ Risk factors

1. Frequently associated with small-cell lung cancer

2. Often presenting symptom of lung cancer

3. Gastrointestinal cancers, thymoma, lymphoma, Hodgkin's disease, bladder and prostate cancer, and sarcoma

4. Certain chemotherapy agents can induce SIADH

   ❏ *Cyclophosphamide*

   ❏ *Vincristine*

   ❏ *Chlorpramide*

   ❏ *Morphine*

   ❏ *Nicotine*

   ❏ *Ethanol*

   ❏ *Cisplatin is associated with SIADH, but mechanism is unknown*

5. Other risk factors

   ❏ *Pulmonary and central nervous system infection*

   ❏ *Neurologic trauma*

❑ *Anesthesia*

❑ *Prolonged intubation*

❑ *Brain tumors*

Approaches to Care

■ Assessment

1. Clinical manifestations

❑ *Early symptoms and signs*

- ☐ Thirst
- ☐ Headache
- ☐ Anorexia
- ☐ Muscle cramps
- ☐ Lethargy

❑ *Late symptoms and signs*

- ☐ Nausea, vomiting
- ☐ Weight gain without edema
- ☐ Hyporeflexia
- ☐ Confusion
- ☐ Oliguria
- ☐ Seizures
- ☐ Coma

2. Diagnostic measures

❑ *Blood and urine chemistries confirm diagnosis*

☐ Serum sodium	<130 mEq/l
☐ Plasma osmolality	<280 mOsm/kg
☐ Urine osmolality	>330 mOsm/kg
☐ Urine sodium	>20 mEq/l

❏ *Water load test can be done by administering specific amount of water and measuring urine output, osmolality, and specific gravity; this is not done if patient is symptomatic or serum sodium is less than 125 mEq/l*

▇ Interventions

1. **Measures are dependent on severity of syndrome and patient's general condition**

2. **If possible, initiate systemic chemotherapy immediately**

3. **Tumor control is only truly effective measure to reverse tumor-induced ectopic syndrome**

4. **Since most chemotherapy regimens require hydration, control fluid levels carefully**

5. **If hyponatremia is mild to moderate (serum sodium 120–134 mEq/l) and patient is clinically stable, fluid restriction of 800 to 1000 cc/24 hours is effective**

6. **If hyponatremia is severe (serum sodium below 115 mEq/l), and/or patient is unstable, more aggressive intervention is needed**

   ❏ *Restrict fluid to 500 cc/24 hours*

   ❏ *Administer hypertonic 3% saline intravenously*

   ❏ *Give furosemide intravenously*

   ❏ *Once fluid/electrolyte balance and neurologic status are stabilized, begin chemotherapy*

7. **SIADH that persists despite initial therapy may be treated with demeclocycline**
   - ❏ *Inhibits action of ADH*
   - ❏ *Induces reversible diabetes insipidus*
   - ❏ *Absorption is affected by foods high in calcium*
   - ❏ *Should be taken on empty stomach*

8. **Nursing measures**
   - ❏ *Administer and manage chemotherapy*
   - ❏ *Educate patient's family*
   - ❏ *Provide support to patient and family*

9. **Self-care measures**
   - ❏ *Restrict fluid*
   - ❏ *Measure intake and output*
   - ❏ *Recognize signs of hyponatremia*
   - ❏ *Know when to contact physician*

10. **If untreated, SIADH can lead to seizure, coma, and death**

11. **Overall prognosis is related to underlying cause and effectiveness of therapy directed toward it**

Suggested Readings

1. Dietz KA, Flaherty AM: Oncologic emergencies. In Groenwald SL, Frogge MH, Goodman M, Yarbro CH (eds.): *Cancer Nursing: Principles and Practice* (3rd ed.). Boston: Jones and Bartlett, 1993, pp. 824–829.

2. Silverman P, Distlehorst CW: Metabolic emergencies in clinical oncology. *Semin Oncol* 16(6):504–515, 1989.

3. Minna JD, Pass H, Glastein EJ, et al: Cancer of the lung. In DeVita VT, Hellman S, Rosenberg SA (eds.): *Cancer Principles and Practice of Oncology* (3rd ed.). Philadelphia: Lippincott, 1989, pp. 591–705.

4. Poe CM, Taylor LM: Syndrome of inappropriate antidiuretic hormone: Assessment and nursing implications. *Oncol Nurs Forum* 16(3):373–382, 1989.

■ 33 ■
Tumor Lysis Syndrome

Overview

■ Complication of cancer therapy that occurs when many rapidly proliferating cells are lysed and release intracellular contents into circulation

■ Results in

1. Hyperuricemia   3. Hyperphosphatemia

2. Hyperkalemia   4. Hypercalcemia

■ Degree of metabolic abnormality depends on renal function

■ Metabolic abnormalities can develop alone or in combination

■ Risk factors

1. Most commonly occurs with high-grade lymphoma or lymphoblastic leukemia

- ❑ *These cells are highly chemosensitive*
- ❑ *These cells rapidly lyse during induction therapy*
- ❑ *Immature lymphoblasts contain abnormally high levels of phosphorous*

2. **Rapidly growing solid tumor that undergoes profound cell destruction**

3. **Acute or chronic myelogenous leukemia**

4. **Non-Hodgkin's lymphoma**

5. **Large tumor burden**

6. **High white blood cell count**

7. **Lymphadenopathy**

8. **Splenomegaly**

9. **Elevated lactate hydrogenase**

Approaches to Care

■ Assessment

1. Clinical manifestations

- ❑ *Early symptoms and signs*
  - ☐ Weakness, paresthesia
  - ☐ Muscle cramps
  - ☐ Nausea, vomiting, diarrhea
  - ☐ Lethargy
- ❑ *Late symptoms and signs*
  - ☐ Ascending flaccid paralysis
  - ☐ Bradycardia, hypotension

□ Oliguria, anuria, edema
□ Hematuria, crystalluria
□ Azotemia, flank pain
□ Carpopedal spasm, laryngospasm
□ Tetany, convulsion

2. Diagnostic measures

❏ *Close monitoring of metabolic parameters enables early identification. Factors are*

□ Potassium   □ Uric acid
□ Phosphorus   □ Blood urea nitrogen
□ Calcium   □ Creatinine levels

❏ *Assess baseline renal function*

■ Interventions

1. Control of hyperuricemia

❏ *Begin allopurinol administration at 600 to 900 mg/day and reduce to half after 3 to 4 days*

2. Urinary alkalinization

❏ *Maintain urine pH ≥7 by addition of 50 to 100 mEq of $NaHCO_3$ to each liter of intravenous fluid*

❏ *Acetazolamide 250 to 500 mg intravenous daily if above measure is ineffective or serum HCO_3 >27 mEq/l*

❏ *Discontinue urinary alkalinization once hyperuricemia is corrected (serum uric acid <10 mg/dl)*

3. Forced diuresis

❏ *Maintain urine flow at more than 150 to 200 ml/hour with infusion of 5% dextrose 0.5NS at 200 ml/hr*

❑ *Initiate low-dose dopamine and diuretics in patients with preexisting evidence of fluid retention (marked edema or ascites) or oliguria*

❑ *Do not insert Foley catheter unless patient has altered mental status or evidence of urinary retention*

4. Maintain fluid balance

❑ *Avoid fluid overload: administer intravenous furosemide (20–100 mg q 4–8 hr) if urine output falls below fluid intake*

❑ *Obtain daily weights*

❑ *Maintain scrupulous records of intake and output*

5. Monitoring of blood chemistries

❑ *Serum electrolytes, blood urea nitrogen, creatinine, uric acid, calcium, phosphorous, magnesium every 6 to 8 hours during the first 72 hours following chemotherapy*

6. Acute hyperkalemia

❑ *Initiate hypertonic glucose and insulin infusion, sodium polystyrene sulfonate (Kayexalate), and furosemide*

7. Hyperphosphatemia

❑ *Initiate hypertonic glucose and insulin infusion, and oral antacids*

8. Resolution occurs when metabolic parameters return to normal

Suggested Readings

1. Dietz KA, Flaherty AM: Oncologic emergencies. In Groenwald SL, Frogge MH, Goodman M, Yarbro CH (eds.): *Cancer Nursing: Principles and Practice* (3rd ed.). Boston: Jones and Bartlett, 1993, pp. 821–824.

2. Simmons ED, Somberg KH: Acute tumor lysis syndrome after intrathecal methotrexate administration. *Cancer* 67:2062–2065, 1991.

3. Marcus SL, Einzig AI: Acute tumor lysis syndrome, prevention and management. In Dutcher JP, Wiernik PH (eds.): *Handbook of Hematologic and Oncologic Emergencies.* New York: Plenum, 1987, pp. 9–16.

4. Silverman P, Distelhorst CW: Metabolic emergencies in clinical oncology. *Semin Oncol* 16(6):504–515, 1989.

PART V

The Care of Individuals with Cancer

Aids-Related Malignancies

Overview

■ Seventy percent of patients with acquired immunodeficiency syndrome (AIDS) develop a malignancy

■ Three most common malignancies in AIDS are

1. **Kaposi's sarcoma (KS)**

   ❏ *More predominant in homosexual and bisexual men*

   ❏ *Mean survival duration is 71.9 weeks*

   ❏ *Etiologic factors may include*
      □ Sexually transmitted agent
      □ Virus (cytomegalovirus has been found in KS lesions)

2. **Non-Hodgkin's lymphoma (NHL)**

   ❏ *French Registry of human immunodeficiency virus–associated tumors reported that 33% of patients with AIDS had NHL*

❏ *Risk factors include*
  ☐ Epstein-Barr virus
  ☐ Therapeutic immunosuppression

3. Central nervous system (CNS) lymphoma

❏ *Most patients are immunocompromised*

❏ *Rare malignancy, accounting for 0.3% to 2% of newly diagnosed lymphomas*

❏ *Cell of origin is same as that causing NHL*

Approaches to Patient Care Kaposi's Sarcoma

■ Assessment

1. Clinical manifestations

❏ *Multicentric skin lesions on any part of body*

❏ *Pigmentation ranges from brown, brown red, and purple to dark red and violet*

❏ *Lesions may be raised nodules or flat and painless*

❏ *Visceral and lymphatic involvement*

❏ *Progressive disease can result in*
  ☐ Enlarging lesions
  ☐ Severe edema due to compromised lymphatic drainage and blood circulation
  ☐ Protein-losing enteropathy due to gastrointestinal involvement
  ☐ Respiratory distress due to lung involvement

2. Diagnostic measures

❏ *Self-observation of cutaneous lesions*
❏ *Biopsy suspicious lesions*
❏ *Histologic examination confirms diagnosis*

■ Interventions

1. Treatment is complex

❏ *Need to control tumor without exacerbating immunodeficiency*

❏ *Radiation therapy for local control of lesions*

❏ *Systemic chemotherapy has resulted in response rates of 25% to 50%*

❏ *Responders to interferon include*
   ☐ Patients with CD4 counts higher than $200/mm^3$
   ☐ No "B" symptoms (fever, night sweats, weight loss)
   ☐ No prior AIDS diagnosis

2. Nursing care

❏ *Determine patient's risk group and whether KS is first diagnosis*

❏ *Consider psychosocial aspects*

❏ *Aggressively assess potential complications*
   ☐ Side effects from chemotherapy are more severe in AIDS patients
   ☐ If severe jaw pain occurs with first dose of vincristine, discontinue drug

❏ *Realistic goals are necessary because of
manipulative and drug-seeking behavior of
some patients*

Non-Hodgkin's Lymphoma

■ Assessment

1. Clinical manifestations

❏ *Usually presents with advanced disease
involving extranodal sites (CNS, bone
marrow, bowel, and anorectum)*

❏ *Peripheral lymphadenopathy may be absent*

❏ *Majority of patients present with high-grade
lymphoma*

2. Diagnostic measures

❏ *Biopsy specimen determines diagnosis and
classification*

❏ *Staging work-up includes*
  ☐ History, physical examination
  ☐ Laboratory tests
  ☐ Chest x-ray
  ☐ Bone marrow biopsy
  ☐ Lumbar puncture
  ☐ Computed tomographic (CT) scans of chest,
    abdomen, and pelvis

■ Interventions

1. Grade of tumor determines treatment options

❏ *Low-grade tumors are uncommon*

❑ *Intermediate-grade tumors are treated with chemotherapy or radiation therapy*

❑ *High-grade tumors are treated with combination chemotherapy*

2. Nursing care

❑ *Care is same as for those with non–AIDS-related NHL*

❑ *Patients with bulky, high-grade disease are at risk for tumor lysis syndrome, which may occur 24 hours after chemotherapy*

❑ *Patients at risk for tumor lysis syndrome should receive*
   ◻ Vigorous hydration (300–500 ml/hr)
   ◻ Allopurinol intravenously or by mouth
   ◻ Urine output monitored every hour
   ◻ Serum chemistry levels monitored every 6 hours
   ◻ Sodium bicarbonate if ordered

Primary CNS Lymphoma

■ Assessment

1. Clinical manifestations
❑ *Confusion*
❑ *Lethargy*
❑ *Memory loss*
❑ *Alterations in personality and behavior*
❑ *Hemiparesis*
❑ *Aphasia*
❑ *Seizures and focal neurologic symptoms*

2. Diagnostic measures

❏ *CT and magnetic resonance imaging reveal single or multiple discrete lesions*

❏ *Toxoplasmosis titers and VDRL tests rule out toxoplasmosis and syphilis*

■ Interventions

1. Whether or not patient is treated, outcome remains same

❏ *Survival ranges from 1.7 to 5.5 months*

2. Nursing care

❏ *Monitor focal findings, motor incoordination, and cognitive deficits*

❏ *Establish safe environment in acute and home setting*

❏ *Provide emotional support to patient and family*

❏ *Plans may be needed for skilled nursing care facility*

❏ *If patient is legally incompetent, legal guardian must be appointed*

Suggested Readings

1. Moran T: AIDS-related malignancies. In Groenwald SL, Frogge MH, Goodman M, Yarbro CH (eds.): *Cancer Nursing: Principles and Practice* (3rd ed.). Boston: Jones and Bartlett, 1993, pp. 861–876.

2. Karp JE, Groopman JE, Broder S: Cancer in AIDS.

In DeVita VT, Hellman S, Rosenberg SA (eds.):
Cancer: Principles and Practice of Oncology (4th ed.).
Philadelphia: JB Lippincott, 1993, pp. 2093–2110.

3. Stanley H, Fluetsch-Bloom M, Bunce-Clyma M:
   HIV-related non-Hodgkin's lymphoma. *Oncol Nurs
   Forum* 18:875–880, 1991.

4. Jacob JL, Baird BF, Haller S, et al: AIDS-related
   Kaposi's sarcoma: Concepts of care. *Semin Oncol
   Nurs* 5:263–275, 1989.

■ 35 ■
Bladder Cancer

Overview

■ Second most common urologic cancer after prostate cancer

■ Occurs in males more frequently than females and has a higher incidence in white men over 50 years of age

■ Risk factors include

1. Cigarette smoking

2. Occupational exposure to industrial chemicals

3. Exposure to schistosomiasis (rare in U.S.)

4. Long-term exposure to cyclophosphamide and pelvic irradiation

■ Approximately 90% are transitional cell carcinoma

■ **Grading of bladder tumors helps to predict recurrence (i.e., low-grade have slower growth rate and better prognosis)**

■ **Five-year survival ranges from 87% for those with localized disease to 9% for those with distant metastasis**

Approaches to Care

■ **Assessment**

1. Clinical manifestations

❑ *Gross hematuria*
❑ *Dysuria*
❑ *Urinary frequency, urgency, and burning*
❑ *Decrease in urinary stream*
❑ *Flank, rectal, back, or suprapubic pain*

2. Diagnostic measures

❑ *Intravenous pyelogram (excretory urogram)*

❑ *Cystoscopy provides view of tumor, biopsies, and bladder washings for cytology and flow cytometry*

❑ *CT scan, bone scan, and chest x-ray*

❑ *Serum chemistries*

■ **Interventions**

1. Treatment selection depends on stage and grade of tumor

❑ Carcinoma in situ *treatment options are*
  □ Transurethral resection

- ☐ Therapeutic cystoscopy followed by intravesical thiotepa, Calmette-Guérin bacillus, or doxorubicin
- ☐ Radical cystectomy with urinary diversion

❏ Superficial, low-grade tumors
  - ☐ More than 70% of patients present with superficial tumors
  - ☐ Treatment options are
    - Transurethral surgery with resection and fulguration
    - Laser therapy
    - Partial cystectomy, which preserves bladder and male erectile function

❏ *Treatment options for* invasive tumors *include*
  - ☐ Radiation alone or in combination with chemotherapy for nonsurgical candidates
  - ☐ Radical cystectomy with urinary diversion with or without pelvic lymph node dissection
  - ☐ Combination chemotherapy for metastatic disease

❏ *Types of urinary diversion*
  - ☐ Ileal conduit
  - ☐ Loop stoma
  - ☐ Continent urinary diversion allows patient to control voiding and urinary reflux after cystectomy
    - Kock pouch
    - Indiana reservoir

2. Sexual dysfunctions due to radical cystectomy

❏ *Body image affected by stoma and appliance*

❏ *Penile prosthesis may help erectile impotence*

❏ *Intercourse is restricted in women and clitoral sensation may be altered*

3. Nursing care involves

❏ *Preoperative selection of stoma site and teaching self-catheterization*

❏ *Postoperative care depends on method of urinary diversion or bladder substitution*

❏ *Urinary diversion with ileal conduit*
  ☐ Assess viability of stoma
  ☐ Appliance must be worn at all times
    ▪ Pouch should adhere for 3 days before changing
  ☐ Good skin care is essential

❏ *Continent urinary diversion*
  ☐ Produces much mucus and needs regular irrigation in early postoperative period; mucus decreases over time
  ☐ No appliance necessary
  ☐ Patient teaching focuses on self-catheterization of pouch; stoma care; and care of catheter

Suggested Readings

1. Lind J, Kravitz K, Greig B: Urologic and male genital malignancies. In Groenwald SL, Frogge MH, Goodman M, Yarbro CH (eds.): *Cancer Nursing: Principles and Practice* (3rd ed.). Boston: Jones and Bartlett, 1993, pp. 1258–1315.

2. Hossan E, Striegel A: Carcinoma of the bladder. *Semin Oncol Nurs* 9:252–266, 1993.

3. Razor B: Continent urinary reservoirs. *Semin Oncol Nurs* 9:272–285, 1993.

■ 36 ■
Bone Sarcomas

Overview

■ Two thousand new cases of bone cancer are diagnosed annually

■ Risk factors

1. Family history

2. Paget's disease

3. Skeletal maldevelopment

■ The most common bone tumors are

1. Osteosarcoma (osteogenic sarcoma)

- ❑ *Most common osseous malignant bone tumor*

- ❑ *Greatest incidence between 10 and 25 years of age*

- ❑ *Twice incidence in men as in women*

- ❑ *Incidence increased in adults with Paget's disease*

- *Most common sites are distal end of femur, proximal end of tibia, and proximal end of humerus*

- *Metastasizes primarily to lungs*

- *Five-year survival rates are low (10%–20%)*

2. Chondrosarcoma

- *Occurs between 30 and 60 years of age and among males*

- *Associated with syndromes of skeletal maldevelopment*

- *Most frequent sites are pelvic bone, long bones, scapula, and ribs*

- *Most remain localized and slow growing*

- *If metastasis occurs, it is usually to lungs*

3. Ewing's sarcoma

- *Accounts for 5% of all malignant bone tumors*

- *Eighty percent are diagnosed in individuals younger than 30 years of age, and 66% more males are affected than females*

- *Commonly located in pelvis and diaphyseal or metadiaphyseal regions of long bones*

- *Metastasis may be present in nearly 20% of individuals at diagnosis*

4. Metastatic bone tumors

❏ *Primary tumors that metastasize to bone include*

☐ Lung ☐ Gastric
☐ Breast ☐ Colon
☐ Prostate ☐ Pancreatic
☐ Kidney ☐ Testicular
☐ Thyroid

❏ *More common sites of metastases include*

☐ Spine ☐ Pelvis
☐ Ribs

Approaches to Patient Care

■ Osteosarcoma

1. Assessment

❏ *Clinical manifestions*

☐ Typically presents as pain and a mass

☐ Pain is more severe at night

☐ Limb becomes swollen with dilated superficial veins

☐ Weight loss and anemia may be seen

☐ Pathologic fractures may occur

❏ *Diagnostic measures*

☐ Elevation in serum alkaline phosphatase level is common

☐ Bone scans

☐ Arteriography

☐ CT

☐ Fluoroscopy

- ☐ MRI
- ☐ Biopsy
- ☐ CT of chest and regional nodes for metastatic disease

2. Treatment

- ❏ *Chemotherapy*
  - ☐ Adjuvant chemotherapy after surgery significantly prolongs disease-free interval
  - ☐ Chemotherapy protocols include doxorubicin, high-dose cyclophosphamide, ifosfamide, cisplatin, or high-dose methotrexate with leucovorin rescue; drugs are given intravenously or intraarterially
  - ☐ Preoperative chemotherapy effectiveness is assessed at time of tumor resection
  - ☐ If there is high degree of tumor necrosis, chemotherapy is continued postoperatively
  - ☐ The greater the necrosis, the greater the survival
  - ☐ Improved response with chemotherapy has sparked interest in limb salvage surgery

- ❏ *Surgery*
  - ☐ Amputations are indicated for patients with large, invasive tumors of extremities
    - ■ Types
      - *Immediate fitting prosthesis*
        - Rigid dressing and cast are applied to stump at time of surgery
        - Socket on distal end of cast attaches to prosthetic unit

Delayed fitting

> Individual fitted with temporary or intermediate prosthesis at approximately 3 to 6 weeks

> Ambulation with weight-bearing is encouraged

> Three months after surgery, individual is fitted with permanent prosthesis

Hemipelvectomy

- Phantom limb pain

> *Thirty-five percent of patients experience phantom limb pain*

> *Severe cramping, throbbing, or burning pain in various areas of amputated limb*

> *Occurs for 1 to 4 weeks after surgery*

> *May be triggered by fatigue, excitement, sickness, weather change, stress*

> *Incidence is greater when amputation site is more proximal*

> *Pain worsens over time for 5% to 10% of amputees*

- Resection of pulmonary metastases with follow-up chemotherapy has resulted in increased survival

- Reconstruction techniques after bone resection

> *Arthrodesis* (fusion)

> *Arthroplasty* (bone allograft or metallic implant)

> *Allograft* (bone graft to provide scaffold for new host bone to grow into)

❏ *Radiation is reserved for palliation of inoperable tumors*

■ Chondrosarcoma

1. Assessment

❑ *Clinical manifestations*

☐ Medical advice is usually sought for slow-growing mass with intermittent dull, aching pain at tumor site

☐ May be a firm enlargement over affected area

☐ Joints may be swollen and exhibit restricted motion

❑ *Diagnostic measures*

☐ Bone scan

☐ Arteriography

☐ CT

☐ Fluoroscopy

☐ MRI

☐ Biopsy

☐ CT of chest and regional nodes for metastatic disease

2. Treatment

❑ *If tumor is of central origin and has not extended through cortex, wide resection and reconstruction are considered*

❑ *Limb salvage surgery or amputation are options*

❑ *Chondrosarcomas are generally avascular; consequently, intravenous chemotherapy is not usually beneficial*

❑ *Radiation has limited effectiveness*

■ Ewing's sarcoma

1. Assessment

❏ *Clinical manifestations*

   ☐ Examination usually reveals palpable and tender mass

   ☐ Temperature may be increased over the mass and small superficial blood vessels may be visible

   ☐ Individual frequently has history of pain that has become increasingly severe

   ☐ Patients often present with fever and anemia

❏ *Diagnostic measures*

   ☐ Patients may present with high erythrocyte sedimentation rates and leukocytosis, indicating aggressive disease

   ☐ Radiographic studies of the bone

2. Treatment

❏ *Radiation or surgery, or both, in combination with chemotherapy is treatment of choice*

❏ *Ewing's sarcoma is radiosensitive and responds well to variety of antineoplastic agents*

   ☐ Ifosfamide   ☐ Vincristine
   ☐ Actinomycin D   ☐ Cyclophosphamide
   ☐ Doxorubicin

❏ *Surgery combined with radiotherapy improves local control rate and can decrease need for extremely high radiation doses*

❏ *Limb salvage and amputation are both options*

■ Metastatic bone tumors

1. Assessment

❏ *Clinical manifestations*

  ☐ Initial presentation may include

  ■ Complaints of dull, aching bone pain that increases steadily as day progresses, and is worse at night

  ■ Tumor weakens bone and can result in pathologic fracture

  ■ Pain, both local and leg pain, is most often seen in spine metastases

  ■ Neurologic dysfunction can precede pain in lesions of thoracic spine (e.g., heavy limb sensation, leg buckling)

  ■ Tenderness or warmth, or both, over lesion may be found on physical examination

❏ *Diagnostic measures*

  ☐ Conventional radiography

  ☐ Bone scan

  ☐ Biopsy is not necessary if appearance of lesion is consistent with known primary tumor

  ☐ Biopsy is indicated in absence of known or suspected primary tumor

  ☐ Hypercalcemia in presence of normal alkaline phosphatase level is associated with breast carcinoma

  ☐ Elevations of serum acid phosphatase occur with prostatic cancer

  ☐ Additional imaging with MRI, CT, or myelogram may be required

2. Treatment

❏ *Surgery*

  ☐ Goals

  - Augment material strength of bone, increasing resistance to fracture

  - Improve functional use of the part

  - Resume ambulatory status

  - Even a bedridden patient with metastatic carcinoma and a femur fracture would benefit from surgery because of pain relief and increased mobility

  - Prophylactic pinning of impending pathologic hip fracture reduces complications

  ☐ Indications for surgical intervention of metastatic spinal disease

  - Intractable pain unresponsive to nonoperative management

  - Progressive neurologic changes during or after radiotherapy

  - Presence of radioresistant tumor

  - Decompression of neural element, or spinal instability

❏ *Radiation*

  ☐ Goals

  - Shrink tumor to facilitate surgical intervention

  - Palliate pain

  - Postoperatively to kill tumor cells and allow surgical implant to maintain anatomic alignment

❑ *Chemotherapy*
  ☐ May be used to reduce tumor cell mass

❑ *Nursing care*
  ☐ Stump care
    ▪ Elevate stump for 24 hours after surgery to prevent edema
    ▪ Patient should lie in prone position 3 to 4 times per day to prevent joint contractures
    ▪ Initiate exercises to maintain muscle tone and prevent edema, joint contractures, and muscle atrophy on first postoperative day
    ▪ Wrap stump with elastic bandages or stump shrinkers
    ▪ Patient should dangle at side of bed and transfer to chair as tolerated
    ▪ Patient should begin crutch walking as soon as possible
    ▪ Sutures or staples will be removed approximately 2 weeks after surgery
    ▪ Wash stump and prosthesis with mild soap and water
    ▪ Inspect stump daily for redness, blisters, or abrasions
    ▪ Patient sees prosthetist every 4 to 6 weeks for first postoperative year
  ☐ Phantom limb sensation
    ▪ Apply heat to stump
    ▪ Apply pressure with elastic bandages
    ▪ Administer tranquilizers, muscle relaxants, or local anesthesia
    ▪ Recommend psychotherapy and behavioral therapy

- Suggest hypnosis, nerve blocks, sympathectomy cordotomy, acupuncture, biofeedback, and transcutaneous nerve stimulation
□ Posthemipelvectomy care
  - Mobilization usually begins on second or third postoperative day
  - Permanent prosthesis may be fitted within 12 weeks
  - Bucket prosthesis is fabricated to facilitate sitting in absence of ischium

Suggested Readings

1. Piasecki PA: Bone and soft tissue sarcoma. In Groenwald SL, Frogge MH, Goodman M, Yarbro CH (eds.): *Cancer Nursing: Principles and Practice* (3rd ed.). Boston: Jones and Bartlett, 1993, pp. 877–902.

2. Mazanet R, Antman K: Sarcomas of soft tissue and bone. *Cancer* 68:463–473, 1991.

3. Piasecki P: The nursing role in limb salvage surgery. *Nurs Clin North Am* 26:33–41, 1991.

4. Williamson V: Amputation of the lower extremity: An overview. *Orthop Nurs* 11:55–65, 1992.

▪ 37 ▪
Breast Cancer

Overview

■ Leading cause of death in women 40 to 44 years of age

■ Incidence in U.S. is 1 in 9 women; incidence varies across the country

■ More than 70% of breast cancers occur in women 50 years of age and older

■ Second leading cause of cancer deaths in women; lung cancer is first

■ Risk factors

1. Primary risk factors
   - ❏ *Female gender*
   - ❏ *Older than 50 years*
   - ❏ *Native of North America or northern Europe*

❏ *Family history*
  ☐ Previous breast cancer
  ☐ Breast cancer in two or more first-degree relatives
  ☐ Bilateral or premenopausal breast cancer in first-degree relative

2. Secondary risk factors

❏ *Postmenopausal obesity*

❏ *Menarche before age 12 years; menopause after age 55*

❏ *First full-term pregnancy after age 35*

❏ *Use of oral contraceptives for more than 6 years before age 20*

❏ *Ionizing radiation exposure to chest before age 35*

❏ *Benign breast disease*

3. Other risk factors

❏ *Nulliparity*

❏ *Ingestion of more than two alcoholic drinks per day*

❏ *High-fat diet*

▧ Types of breast tumors

1. Forty-eight percent of all breast cancers are adenocarcinomas located in upper outer quadrant of breast

2. Infiltrating ductal carcinoma

❏ *Prominent lump; stony hardness on palpation*
❏ *Primarily affects women in early fifties*
❏ *Ten-year survival 50% to 60%*

3. Invasive lobular carcinoma

❏ *Multicentric bilaterality in 30% of patients*
❏ *Accounts for 5% to 10% of all breast cancers*
❏ *Primarily affects women in their fifties*
❏ *Ten-year survival is 50% to 60%*

4. Tubular carcinoma

❏ *Uncommon; 2% of all breast cancers*

❏ *Well-differentiated adenocarcinoma*

❏ *Primarily affects women ≥55 years*

❏ *Microcalcification often present, facilitating early detection on mammography*

5. Medullary carcinomas

❏ *Account for 5% to 7% of all breast cancers*

❏ *Primarily affects women younger than 55 years*

❏ *Lymph node involvement in 40% at diagnosis*

❏ *Well circumscribed, rapid growth rate, bilaterality*

6. Mucinous (colloid) carcinomas

❏ *Uncommon; 3% of all breast cancers*

❏ *Primarily affects women 60 to 70 years old*

❏ *Characterized by large pools of mucin with small islands of tumor cells*

❏ *Slow growing, bulky*

7. Other malignant breast tumors

- ❏ *Sarcomas*
- ❏ *Papillary carcinoma*
- ❏ *Apocrine*
- ❏ *Invasive cribriform*
- ❏ *Paget's disease*

■ Classification and staging of breast cancer

1. Nodal involvement determined only by pathologic evaluation

2. Breast cancer staged clinically on basis of primary tumor characteristics, physical examination of axillary nodes, and presence of distant metastases

- ❏ Stage I *is localized disease only*

- ❏ Stage II *has axillary nodal involvement on pathology*

- ❏ Stage III *is more advanced locoregional disease with no distant metastasis*

- ❏ Stage IV *involves presence of distant metastasis*

Approaches to Patient Care

■ Assessment

1. Clinical manifestations of malignant disease

- ❏ *Boundaries of mass not distinct*

- ❏ *Lack of mobility of mass due to tumor infiltration into adjacent tissues*

- ❏ *Pain not common; may be present in advanced disease*

- ❏ *Pink or bloody, spontaneous, unilateral discharge from nipples*

- ❏ *Elevation or retraction of nipples resulting from tumor fixation or infiltration into underlying tissues*

- ❏ *Skin dimpling or retraction possibly caused by invasion of suspensory ligaments and fixation to chest wall*

- ❏ *Heat and erythema may signify inflammatory breast carcinoma*

- ❏ *Skin edema (peau d'orange) may be caused by tumor invasion and obstruction of dermal lymphatics*

- ❏ *Ulceration of skin with secondary infection*

- ❏ *Isolated skin nodules signify tumor invasion of blood vessels and lymphatics*

- ❏ *Ulceration or scaly skin at nipple may indicate Paget's disease*

- ❏ *May also include, or may be limited to, signs of local or distant metastatic disease*

2. Diagnostic procedures

❏ *Screening mammogram*

- ☐ Used for routine observation of breast tissue in asymptomatic women

- ☐ Goal is to detect malignancy before it becomes clinically apparent

- ☐ Recommended every 1 to 2 years for women 40 to 49; yearly for women 50 years or older

❏ *Diagnostic mammogram*

- ☐ Done when patient reports specific symptoms, when clinical findings are suspicious, or when screening mammogram reveals abnormality

- ☐ Information learned on diagnostic mammography may prevent need for open biopsy

❏ *Sonogram or ultrasound*

- ☐ Used to determine whether lesion is solid or cystic

- ☐ Sensitivity and specificity not equal to mammograms; therefore not used for screening purposes

❏ *MRI*

- ☐ May allow earlier detection because it can determine smaller lesions and finer detail

- ☐ Complement to mammography and clinical examination in distinguishing benign from malignant lesions and avoiding benign biopsy

❏ *Fine-needle aspiration*
  □ Used when abnormality is known to be solid or to determine whether lump is cyst
  □ Surgical biopsy may still be necessary for lesion that is not malignant on histologic study but remains clinically suspicious

❏ *Stereotactic needle-guided biopsy*
  □ Most frequently used to target and identify nonpalpable lesions detected on mammography
  □ Permits diagnosis of benign disease without trauma or scarring related to open biopsy

❏ *Wire localization biopsy*
  □ Primarily used to assist in location of nonpalpable lesions for excisional biopsy

❏ *Open biopsy*
  □ Objective to remove lump or identified area along with small amount of surrounding normal tissue
  □ Reasons for excisional biopsy
    ▪ Sonogram reveals solid lesion
    ▪ Insufficient findings on histologic or cytologic studies, or both
    ▪ Suspicious findings on mammogram or on clinical examination
    ▪ Patient with probable low-risk lesion requests biopsy to alleviate anxiety

▣ Interventions

1. **Most women with stage I and stage II breast cancer with positive or negative nodes can be treated by breast conservation procedures**

❏ *Lumpectomy*
❏ *Partial mastectomy*
❏ *Segmental resection*
❏ *Quadrantectomy and breast irradiation*

2. **Invasive breast cancer requires level I and II axillary node dissection, depending on whether axillary nodes are tumor-positive**

3. **Modified radical mastectomy is indicated for**

   ❏ *Larger tumors*

   ❏ *Multicentric disease*

   ❏ *When cosmesis is otherwise not achievable*

   ❏ *Women who prefer not to undergo radiation therapy*

   ❏ *Involves removal of all breast tissue and nipple areola complex and level I and II axillary node dissection*

   ❏ *May also be used as definitive treatment after local recurrence in those who fail conservative surgery and radiation therapy*

4. **Carcinoma in situ is being detected more often by mammography**

   ❏ *Lobular carcinoma usually discovered during removal of benign tumor*
   ◻ Tends to be bilateral and multicentric
   ◻ If not treated there is 50% chance that invasive breast cancer will develop in either breast

- ☐ Management includes
  - ■ Observation with annual mammography and frequent physical examination
  - ■ Ipsilateral mastectomy with contralateral biopsy
  - ■ Bilateral mastectomy with immediate or delayed reconstruction
- ❏ *Intraductal carcinoma generally presents as clustered microcalcifications on mammography*
  - ☐ Rarely carries risk of axillary node involvement
  - ☐ Treatment options
    - ■ Total mastectomy with low axillary dissection
    - ■ Wide excision followed by radiation
    - ■ Wide excision alone with tumor-free margins
  - ☐ Invasive carcinoma develops in 30% to 50% of patients within 10 years when treated with excisional biopsy alone
  - ☐ Total mastectomy and low axillary dissection are recommended as definitive treatment in presence of poor prognostic indicators such as ploidy and high nuclear grade

5. **Radiation treatment for localized breast cancer now standard treatment, making breast conservation realistic possibility**

- ❏ *Conservative surgery plus radiation now considered preferable to mastectomy in most women*
  - ☐ Criteria for selecting patients are feasibility of resecting primary tumor without causing major cosmetic deformity and likelihood of tumor recurrence in breast

❑ *Radiation more successful when all gross disease has been resected*

❑ *When chemotherapy is also used, radiation is usually given concurrently to minimize local recurrence*

6. Adjuvant systemic therapy for

❑ *Early stage I and stage II breast cancer*

☐ Metastatic disease occurs in 30% to 50% of women with node-negative breast cancer

☐ Systemic chemotherapy is indicated for women with large, poorly differentiated tumors

☐ Annual odds of tumor recurrence reduced to approximately 30% by combination chemotherapy

☐ Potential drug combinations

   ▪ Methotrexate, followed in 1 hour by 5-fluorouracil (M-F); leucovorin calcium (L) is given beginning 24 hours after administration of methotrexate

   Regimen given on days 1 and 8, every 28 days, for 6 cycles

   Appears to be less toxic in terms of myelosuppression and hair loss; does not have the leukemogenic potential of alkylating agent–containing regimen

   ▪ Cyclophosphamide, methotrexate, and 5-fluorouracil (CMF)

   Methotrexates and 5-fluorouracil given on days 1 and 8; cyclophosphamide given orally for 14 days; CMF combination administered every 28 days for 6 cycles

Myelosuppression, hair loss, and gonadal dysfunction more pronounced with this regimen because cyclophosphamide is alkylating agent

More effective than M-F+L regimen for treatment of premenopausal women; this may be due to alkylating agent

- Doxorubicin and cyclophosphamide, given in standard doses every 3 weeks for 4 cycles

  Treatment option for women with high-risk node-negative disease or with node-positive disease

  Dose-intensive regimens may be employed, using colony-simulating factors to boost marrow recovery

- Treatment with tamoxifen may be appropriate based on patient age (>50 yr) and estrogen receptor status

  May be given alone or in combination chemotherapy

- Goserelin acetate (luteinizing hormone–releasing hormone antagonist), with or without tamoxifen and chemotherapy, may be used to treat premenopausal women with estrogen receptor-positive, node-positive disease

❏ *Locally advanced (stage III) breast cancer*
  ☐ More likely to metastasize to distant sites; larger primary tumor and greater number of histologically positive lymph nodes, greater risk of metastasis
    - Distant metastasis is presumed present at diagnosis

□ Treatment of choice is modified radical mastectomy

□ Clinical characteristics include large or unresectable primary tumors, fixed axillary nodes, internal mammary node involvement, and presence of classic inflammatory carcinoma

□ Potential treatment options

- Primary chemotherapy to evaluate tumor's in vivo response to drug combination; if significant tumor reduction occurs, surgery may be indicated, followed by chemotherapy and radiation therapy

- High-dose chemotherapy with autologous bone marrow rescue and support with hematopoietic growth factor is currently treatment option for women with high-risk advanced disease

7. Chemotherapy

❏ *Premenopausal women often experience symptoms of menopause because of effects of drugs on ovarian function*

□ Less subjective sexual desire and arousability
□ Vaginal dryness
□ Vulvar or vaginal soreness
□ Light spotting after intercourse
□ Hot flashes or night sweats
□ Sleep disturbances

❏ *Measures to minimize symptoms of ovarian failure*

□ Lower thermostat in home, especially in sleeping area

□ Avoid highly seasoned foods

□ Avoid caffeine and alcohol

- ☐ Dress in loose-fitting clothing and in layers
- ☐ Take vitamin E 800 international units per day or Bellergal-S 1 tablet twice daily or use clonidine patch, 0.1 to 0.2 mg

❏ *Some women experience weight gain and may require nutritional counselling*

❏ *Fatigue is common complaint; advise patient to rest and begin regular exercise program such as walking, aerobics, or water aerobics*

❏ *Nausea and vomiting are predictable based on type of chemotherapy or hormone therapy; give prophylactic treatment with antiemetics such as ondansetron, dexamethasone, and lorazepam in combination*

❏ *High doses of doxorubicin and cyclophosphamide cause hair loss, with total hair loss occurring 17 to 21 days after first treatment; CMF treatment causes more gradual thinning over the six-course treatment and may not require patient to use wig*

8. Radiation

❏ *Generally begins 3 to 4 weeks after chemotherapy*

❏ *Side effects include fatigue and some nausea; primary side effects are skin changes and arm swelling*
- ☐ Skin reactions occur in all patients and include itching, dryness, scaling, redness, and tenderness
  - ▪ Dry desquamation can progress to moist desquamation with infection

❏ *If chemotherapy is being given along with radiation, chemotherapy should be held until skin heals*

9. Breast reconstruction

❏ *Ideal candidate is woman with early-stage disease, no nodal involvement, and low-risk factors for recurrence*

❏ *Women who are pregnant or breastfeeding, or who have tissue abnormalities, infection, lupus, scleroderma, or uncontrolled diabetes are not candidates*

❏ *Those with radiation damage, vascularization problems, or who have inadequate tissue available are not eligible*

❏ *Procedures*

  ☐ Silicone implants are used when there is adequate skin for coverage after mastectomy

   ▪ Ideal candidate is small-breasted and has minimum of ptosis on contralateral breast

   ▪ Incision is made in previous scar and pocket is made beneath chest wall muscles where silicone implant will be placed

   ▪ Complications

Contracture	*Infection*
Hematoma	*Flap necrosis*

  ☐ Saline tissue expanders are used when there is inadequate supply of skin after mastectomy or when the breast is large and/or ptotic

   ▪ Expander is placed behind muscles of chest wall using lines of mastectomy incision

- Filling port is injected with saline over 6 to 8 weeks until device is overinflated by 50%; it is left overinflated for several months to allow for stretching and more natural contour

- Expander is removed after several months and replaced with permanent prosthesis

☐ Latissimus dorsi flap is used when adequate skin is not available at mastectomy site and/or if additional tissue is needed to fill supraclavicular hollow and create anterior axillary fold after radical mastectomy

☐ Transverse rectus abdominis muscle flap, or "tummy tuck"

- Incision is made over lower abdomen; abdominal muscle and fat are tunneled under abdominal skin to mastectomy site

- Possible complications include hernia at donor site and flap necrosis

- Obese patients, patients with circulatory problems, smokers, and patients over 65 are not candidates

☐ Use of free flap entails removal of skin and fat from buttocks or lower abdomen and grafting them to mastectomy site

- Main complication is failure to maintain sufficient perfusion during postoperative period; flap death will occur within 6 hours if flow is interrupted and cannot be sustained

☐ Nipple areolar construction by using tissue from opposite breast or from like tissue on inner thigh or postauricular area

- Tattooing may be necessary to darken skin

■ Raising and folding skin over itself creates more natural nipple projection, called skate flap

10. Breast cancer in men

❑ *Similar to breast cancer in women in terms of epidemiology, natural history, treatment options, and response to treatment*

❑ *Occurs most commonly in men aged 50 to 70; most are estrogen receptor–positive*

❑ *Typically presents as infiltrating ductal carcinoma, fixed to underlying fascia and skin; nipple retraction and bloody discharge may be present*

☐ Because it is usually first diagnosed at advanced stage, prognosis is generally poor

❑ *Treatment is usually by modified radical mastectomy*

❑ *Hormonal manipulation is indicated using tamoxifen, aminoglutethimide, or orchiectomy, unless disease is life-threatening or aggressive, indicating use of chemotherapy*

11. Metastatic breast cancer

❑ *Present at clinical diagnosis in approximately 10% of women diagnosed with breast cancer*

❑ *Disease will metastasize in 30% to 40% of women diagnosed and treated for potentially curable breast cancer, and these women will die of disease*

❑ *Relapse occurs within 2 years of diagnosis in most patients*

❏ *Median survival for patients with stage IV disease is 2 to 3 years*

❏ *Metastases most commonly occur to bone, specifically spine, ribs, and proximal long bones*
  ☐ Pathologic fractures may occur despite efforts to protect weakened bone

❏ *Early symptoms of liver involvement include loss of appetite and abnormal results on liver function tests*

❏ *Pulmonary involvement may be manifested as nonproductive cough or shortness of breath*
  ☐ Lymphangitic pulmonary spread is ominous sign of rapidly progressing disease
  ☐ Pleural effusions may progress slowly over time and may respond temporarily to drainage and sclerosing

❏ *Metastasis to brain or meningeal carcinomatosis may present as seizures or cranial nerve palsies*

❏ *Management*
  ☐ Judicious use of both local and systemic measures to palliate symptoms and improve patient's quality of life
  ☐ Initial choice of therapy is one that is least toxic with highest response rate
  ☐ Chemotherapy
    ▪ Candidates include those women whose disease is hormone-receptor negative, those who are refractory to hormone therapy, or those with aggressive disease in liver or pulmonary system

- Most chemotherapy regimens include some combination of methotrexate, 5-fluorouracil, cyclophosphamide, doxorubicin, or taxol mitoxantrone every 3 to 4 weeks

- After response to treatment is seen, interval between treatments can be lengthened; therapeutic benefit not compromised, but cost and inconvenience to patient are decreased

□ Endocrine therapy

- Important for treatment of metastatic disease that is estrogen-receptor–positive

- Steroid hormones promote tumor growth in hormonally dependent breast cancer; therefore, surgical removal of hormone source or medical manipulation of hormone balance results in significant tumor regression, but not cure

- Estrogen therapy

  In about 35% of patients, pharmacologic doses of estrogens (diethylstilbestrol 5 mg, 2–3 times/day) can result in objective remission

  Therapy may cause nausea and vomiting for few days; fluid retention may require diuretics

  Women who initially respond to estrogen therapy and then fail may benefit from estrogen withdrawal

  Estrogen withdrawal may cause uterine bleeding

- Androgen therapy

  Most effective in women who are 5 years postmenopause

Indicated for treatment of soft-tissue or bone metastases

Therapeutic effect exerted through androgen's opposition of endogenous estrogens

Side effects of fluoxymesterone include fluid retention, erythrocytosis, and masculinization

Patient may experience increased libido, hair loss, amenorrhea, nausea, and anorexia

- Progestin therapy

  Megestrol acetate is progesterone agent that is tolerated as well as tamoxifen and has comparable efficacy

  Side effects of megestrol acetate include weight gain, hot flashes, vaginal bleeding, hypercalcemia, tumor flare, and thrombophlebitis

- Corticosteroid therapy

  Corticosteroids (prednisone) in pharmacologic doses can suppress pituitary adrenocorticotropic hormone secretion, thereby opposing estrogen-progesterone secretion from adrenals

  Steroids are often used as adjunct radiotherapy in cerebral metastasis, in chemotherapy for liver and lung metastasis, and in management of hypercalcemia

  Side effects include bleeding peptic ulcer, muscle weakness, hypertension, infection, edema, glucose intolerance, moon faces, and osteoporosis

- Anti-estrogen therapy

  Compete with estrogen-receptor sites, blocking effect of estrogen on target tissues

  Patients with bone disease may have transient bone pain and hypercalcemia at beginning of therapy; these are usually considered favorable tumor responses

  Tamoxifen, a potent anti-estrogen, is indicated for treatment of both primary and metastatic breast cancer; currently tamoxifen is first-line therapy for postmenopausal women with estrogen receptor–positive tumors

  Side effects of tamoxifen are minimal, including hot flashes, mild nausea, fluid retention and ankle swelling, vaginal cornification, and postmenopausal bleeding

- Oophorectomy

  Generally reserved for women with recurrent or metastatic disease, if disease is not life-threatening at time of recurrence

  Surgical oophorectomy, tamoxifen, or ovarian radiation are equally effective in removing endogenous estrogen sources in premenopausal women and in some perimenopausal women; surgical oophorectomy also may be indicated for women with estrogen receptor–positive tumors

- Secondary endocrine ablation with aminoglutethimide

  Effectively blocks adrenal steroid synthesis and inhibits peripheral conversion of androgens to estrogens

Hydrocortisone replacement needed because of adrenal suppression

Side effects include lethargy and skin rash, which subside if hydrocortisone dose is increased temporarily

❏ *Complications of metastatic disease*

  ☐ Bone metastasis

- Bone pain may occur before skeletal changes are seen on radiography; bone scan is sensitive method to detect metastatic disease

- Metastasis to bone marrow is indicated by anemia, thrombocytopenia, leukocytosis, and immature forms of nucleated red blood cells; serum alkaline phosphatase level and serum calcium level may be increased

- Patients who have back pain should undergo thorough neurologic examination and radiographic evaluation of spine; MRI may determine whether spinal cord compression is present or imminent

- Radiation to symptomatic areas often results in effective pain relief and bone recalcification

- Surgery may stabilize bone by internal fixation or replacement to avoid impending fracture

  ☐ Spinal cord compression

- Constitutes emergency because of potential for paraplegia; pain is usually present for several weeks before other neurologic symptoms develop

- May be secondary to epidural tumor or altered bone alignment due to pathologic fracture

- Imminent compression should be suspected in those with known bone disease; progressive back pain associated with weakness; paresthesias; bowel or bladder dysfunction; or gait disturbances

- MRI should be done as soon as diagnosis is suspected to determine exact level of compression and to identify other occult extradural lesions

- Optimal results and return to ambulation can be accomplished by combined therapy with radiotherapy and corticosteroids

- When spinal cord compression develops and diagnosis of epidural metastasis is in doubt or if patient's neurologic state worsens as radiotherapy progresses, decompression laminectomy may be performed

☐ Brain metastasis and leptomeningeal carcinomatosis

- Brain metastasis occurs in approximately 30% of patients

  Signs include

Headaches	Motor weakness
Seizures	Mental changes
Visual defects	

  Symptoms of brain metastasis can be managed by total-brain irradiation and corticosteroids

■ Leptomeningeal carcinomatosis

Most common signs are

  Headache
  Cranial nerve dysfunction
  Changes in mental status

Treatment is with total-brain irradiation followed by intraventricular-intrathecal chemotherapy, usually through Ommaya reservoir

□ Chronic lymphedema

■ Occurs most commonly in women who have undergone axillary dissection followed by radiation therapy

■ Most often caused by infection and tumor recurrence or tumor enlargement in axilla

■ Management techniques include

Elevation of arm

Use of elastic stockinette

Therapeutic massage

Intermittent compression with extremity pump

Weight loss and weight control may be advised

Suggested Readings

1. Goodman M, Chapman D: Breast cancer. In Groenwald SL, Frogge MH, Goodman M, and Yarbro CH (eds.). *Cancer Nursing: Principles and Practice* (3rd ed.). Boston: Jones and Bartlett, 1993, pp. 903–958.

2. National Institutes of Health Consensus Development Conference Statement: Treatment of Early Stage Breast Cancer. Bethesda, MD: National Institutes of Health, 1990.

3. Bonadonna G: Evolving concepts in the systemic adjuvant treatment of breast cancer. *Cancer Res* 52:2127–2137, 1992.

4. Early Breast Cancer Trialists' Collaborative Group: Systemic Treatment of Early Breast Cancer by Hormonal Cytotoxic or Immune Therapy: Part I and II. *N Engl J. Med* 339:1–15, 71–85, 1992.

∎ 38 ∎
Cancer of the Kidney

Overview

■ Accounts for only 3% of all cancers

■ Occurs most frequently at 50 to 60 years of age

■ Risk factors include

1. Smoking (cigarette, cigar, pipe)

2. Occupational exposure to hydrocarbon, cadmium, asbestos, and lead

3. Analgesic use

■ Common forms of kidney cancer are

1. Renal cell carcinoma, which accounts for 75% to 85% of cases

2. Cancer of renal pelvis

Approaches to Patient Care

■ Assessment

1. Clinical manifestations

❏ *Hematuria*

❏ *Pain*

❏ *Palpable abdominal mass*

❏ *Fever*

❏ *Weight loss*

❏ *Anemia*

❏ *Paraneoplastic syndromes in 30% of presentations*

❏ *30% to 50% of patients have metastasis at diagnosis*

2. Diagnostic measures

❏ *Radiographs of kidney, ureter, and bladder*
❏ *Nephrotomograms*
❏ *Excretory urogram (intravenous pyelogram)*
❏ *Ultrasound*
❏ *CT scan*
❏ *Urinary cytology*
❏ *DNA flow cytometry*

■ Interventions

1. Treatment of renal cell carcinoma includes

❏ *Surgical removal of kidney and tumor thrombus if there is vena caval involvement*

❏ *Regional lymphadenectomy is controversial*

❑ *Interleukin-2 and interferon are under investigation*

❑ *Radiotherapy, surgery, chemotherapy, hormonal therapy, and immunotherapy have been used for advanced disease*

2. **Treatment of cancer of renal pelvis**
   ❑ *Nephroureterectomy is standard treatment*
   ❑ *Use of radiation therapy is controversial*

3. **Preoperative and postoperative nursing care of patient undergoing radical nephrectomy is similar to that of individual undergoing laparotomy**

Suggested Readings

1. Lind J, Kravitz K, Greig B: Urologic and male genital malignancies. In Groenwald SL, Frogge MH, Goodman M, Yarbro CH (eds.): *Cancer Nursing: Principles and Practice* (3rd ed.). Boston: Jones and Bartlett, 1993, pp. 1258–1315.

2. Davis M: Renal cell carcinoma. *Semin Oncol Nurs* 9:267–271, 1993.

▪ 39 ▪
Central Nervous System Cancers

Overview

▪ Involvement of tumor within central nervous system (CNS) as result of primary or metastatic disease is associated with high degree of morbidity and mortality

▪ Increased disease-free intervals, better local control, and longer survival of persons with cancer have resulted in relative increase in incidence of brain metastases from primary sites such as lung, breast, and colon

▪ More than 50% of primary brain tumors are malignant

▪ Approximately 16,700 new primary brain and CNS tumors are diagnosed each year in U.S., with 11,500 deaths

■ Causative factors

1. **Radiation to brain for benign conditions or for acute lymphocytic leukemia**

2. **Immunosuppressive therapy**

3. **Occupational exposure**
   - ❏ *Vinyl chloride*
   - ❏ *Plutonium*
   - ❏ *Petroleum*

■ Types of CNS tumors

1. **Primary brain tumors arise from neuroepithelial cells (glial cells) and are called *gliomas***
   - ❏ *Astrocytomas*
     - □ Incidence greatest in fifth and sixth decades of life
     - □ Largest group of primary brain tumors of one cell type
     - □ Ten percent of all primary brain tumors
     - □ Generally arise in cerebral hemispheres
     - □ Range from well-differentiated to highly malignant
   - ❏ *Oligodendrogliomas*
     - □ Five percent of primary brain tumors
     - □ Usually located in frontal lobe
     - □ Slow growing
     - □ Commonly present as seizure disorder
   - ❏ *Glioblastomas*
     - □ Most common; 60% of primary adult brain tumors

☐ Arise in cerebral hemispheres; predilection for frontal lobe

☐ Occur in fifth and sixth decades of life

☐ Typically grade IV tumor

❏ *Primary malignant lymphomas*

☐ Rare; less than 1% of primary brain tumors

☐ Incidence tripled from 1980s to 1990s

☐ Immunosuppressed individuals at highest risk

2. Spinal cord tumors

❏ *May be primary or metastatic*
❏ *Result in spinal cord compression*

3. Metastatic brain tumors

❏ *Account for 24% of total cancer deaths*

4. Meningeal carcinomatosis from adenocarcinoma of breast, lung, gastrointestinal tract, melanoma, and childhood leukemia occurs in approximately 4% of cases

Approaches to Patient Care

■ Assessment

1. Clinical manifestations

❏ *Caused by increased intracranial pressure (ICP)*

☐ Brain tumors displace components of intracranial cavity because of

- Tumor size
- Cerebral edema
- Obstruction of cerebrospinal fluid (CSF) pathways

- ☐ Clinical manifestations produced by effects of increasing pressure on nerve cells, blood vessels, and dura include
  - Mental changes
  - Papilledema
  - Headache
  - Vomiting
  - Changes in vital signs
- ☐ Prolonged increase in ICP produces nerve cell damage and cell death

❏ *Caused by secondary effects of displacement of brain structures*
  - ☐ Shifting brain tissue causes compression damage, cerebral edema, and ischemia, causing effects that may be irreversible
  - ☐ Two classifications of herniations
    - Supratentorial herniations cause changes in level of consciousness and in ocular, motor, and respiratory signs
    - Infratentorial herniations cause loss of consciousness and changes in cardiac and respiratory signs

❏ *Focal effects*
  - ☐ Caused by direct compression of nerve tissue or destruction and invasion of brain tissues; deficits directly related to affected area of brain
  - ☐ Focal or generalized seizures are major symptoms of brain tumors; first clinical manifestation of disease in many adults

❑ *Patients with metastatic brain tumors commonly have headache first, followed by focal weakness, mental disturbances, and seizures; aphasia and visual abnormalities may also occur*

2. Diagnostic measures

❑ *Document both focal and generalized symptoms*

  □ Examine each symptom with regard to location, onset, and duration (if applicable)

❑ *Take baseline measurement of neurologic function*

❑ *CT views one plane of cranium over a few seconds*

  □ Photographs give exact location and size of nodules

  □ Demonstrates amount of edema surrounding tumor

  □ Less costly than MRI

❑ *MRI allows multiplane imaging*

  □ Provides information regarding histology and pathology of lesions and extent of tissue invasion

  □ Detects deep lesions and cyst formation, amount of edema surrounding tumor, and calcium aggregates

❏ *Positron-emission tomography combines properties of conventional nuclear scanning with physical characteristics of positron-emitting radionuclides*

☐ Provides information about tumor metabolism, bloodflow, and oxygen and glucose use

❏ *Clinical staging based on neurologic signs and symptoms and on results of diagnostic tests*

❏ *Pathologic staging based on results of histopathologic studies, tumor grade, and microscopic evidence of completeness of tumor resection*

■ Treatment

1. Surgery

❏ *Primary treatment*

❏ *In metastatic brain tumors, may be palliative measure to improve quality of life and (possibly) overall survival*

❏ *Factors in evaluating surgical option*

☐ Tumor location
☐ Tumor size
☐ Method of tumor spread
☐ Patient's general condition
☐ Patient's neurologic status

❏ *Goals of surgery*

☐ Primary treatment
☐ Facilitation of nonsurgical therapy
  ■ Partial resection debulks the tumor and relieves symptoms
☐ Treatment of metastatic brain tumors

❏ *Complications*
  ☐ Intracranial bleeding
  ☐ Cerebral edema
  ☐ Water intoxication

❏ *Signs and symptoms of neurosurgery complications*
  ☐ Decreasing level of consciousness
  ☐ Increased ICP
  ☐ Progressive hemiparesis
  ☐ Signs of herniation
  ☐ Seizures

2. Radiosurgery

❏ *Stereotactic radiosurgery is noninvasive technique that delivers single large fraction of ionizing radiation to small, well-defined intracranial target*

❏ *Especially effective in treatment of tumors in or near sensitive target structures*

3. Radiotherapy

❏ *Used for both primary and metastatic disease; response is based on cell type and tissue of origin*

❏ *Corticosteroid therapy may be needed to relieve cerebral swelling and promote improvement of symptoms*

❏ *Presence of hypoxic malignant cells limits effectiveness of radiation therapy*

❏ *Administration of intraoperative radiation may help to shield normal tissue from radiation effects while exposing tumor to maximum radiation effects*

4. Chemotherapy and related drugs

- ❏ *Most chemotherapeutic agents do not cross blood-brain barrier*

- ❏ Nitrosoureas *are drugs that are lipid-soluble and can penetrate blood-brain barrier*

- ❏ *Chemotherapy is indicated for histologic grade III or grade IV tumors*

- ❏ *Intraarterial, intrathecal, and intratumoral drug delivery may circumvent blood-brain barrier*

5. General supportive measures

- ❏ *Prepare family and home environment for patient to be cared for at home*

- ❏ *Cerebral edema*
  - ☐ Corticosteroids are usually prescribed
    - ▪ Reduction of edema may occur over period of hours or days
    - ▪ Less helpful in treatment of acutely increased ICP
  - ☐ Osmotherapy is used to reduce amount of fluid in brain tissue
    - ▪ Hyperosmolar agent such as mannitol is administered intravenously
    - ▪ Fluid intake is restricted

- ❏ *Increased ICP*
  - ☐ Avoid Valsalva's maneuver, isometric muscle contractions, emotional arousal
  - ☐ Elevate head of bed, avoid head rotation, neck flexion and extension
  - ☐ Avoid sneezing, coughing, straining

☐ Avoid hip flexion, prone position

☐ Monitor ICP level

❏ *Seizures*

☐ Provide prophylactic anticonvulsants

☐ Provide safe environment

☐ Prevent harm during seizure activity

☐ Provide skin and oral hygiene following seizure activity

❏ *Personality changes*

☐ Maintain normal function

☐ Maintain orientation with clocks, calendars

☐ Encourage use of remaining cognitive function

☐ Encourage social activities

❏ *Loss of sensation*

☐ Monitor for visual disturbances

☐ Monitor for hearing loss

☐ Maintain orientation

☐ Provide safe environment and clothing

❏ *Disturbances in coordination*

☐ Provide safety devices (bed rails, walker)

☐ Close off stairways

☐ Prepare physical surroundings for safety

❏ *Poor nutrition and hydration*

☐ Prepare small, attractive, frequent meals

☐ Provide dietary supplements

☐ Encourage frequent oral fluids

☐ Use alternative feeding routes, if necessary

❏ *Need for supportive care*
  ☐ Assess roles and family functioning
  ☐ Provide resources
  ☐ Educate and support
  ☐ Prepare for impending death

Suggested Readings

1. Wegmann JA: Central nervous system cancers. In Groenwald SL, Frogge MH, Goodman M, Yarbro CH (eds.). *Cancer Nursing: Principles and Practice* (3rd ed.). Boston: Jones and Bartlett, 1993, pp. 959–983.

2. Gilman S: Advances in neurology. *N Engl J Med* 326:167–176, 1992.

3. Stein DA, Chamberlain MC: Evaluation and management of seizures in the patient with cancer. *Oncology* 5:33–40, 1991.

4. Blaney SM, Balis FM, Poplak DG: Pharmacologic approaches to the treatment of meningeal malignancy. *Oncology* 5:107–127, 1991.

5. Wegmann JA: CNS tumors: Supportive management of the patient and family. *Oncology* 5:109–112, 1991.

▪ 40 ▪
Cervical Cancer

Overview

▪ Approximately 13,500 new cases and 4400 deaths from cervical cancer occurred in 1993 in U.S.

▪ Women over 65 years of age account for 24% of new cases and 40% of deaths

▪ Overall incidence has decreased by 50%

▪ Incidence of carcinoma in situ (CIS) has significantly increased since 1945

1. Over 55,000 new cases diagnosed in 1993

2. Women in their twenties are most often diagnosed with cervical dysplasia

3. Women 30 to 39 years of age are most often diagnosed with CIS

4. Women over 40 years are most often diagnosed with invasive cancer

■ Pap smear, an early detection tool, has resulted in steady decline in incidence of invasive cervical cancer

■ Cervical cancer is significant health problem for women age 65 and over

■ Risk factors

1. Predominantly personal or lifestyle factors

2. Low socioeconomic groups

3. Smoking

4. Early sexual activity (<17 yrs of age)

5. Sexually transmitted infections

6. Higher herpes simplex virus type 2 titers than controls

7. Human papillomavirus (HPV 16 and 18)

8. Multiple sexual partners

9. Spouse whose previous wife had cervical cancer

10. Maternal use of diethylstilbestrol

11. Immunosuppression

12. Multiparity

13. Spouse with cancer of penis

14. African American or Hispanic origin

■ **Certain behaviors may actually lower risk of cervical cancer**

1. Pap smears as recommended
2. Pelvic examinations
3. Barrier contraception
4. Limited number of sexual partners
5. Sex initiated at later age
6. Smoking cessation

■ **Pathophysiology**

1. Progressive disease
2. Begins with neoplastic alteration of cells at squamocolumnar junction
3. Gradually progresses to involve full thickness of epithelium
4. Preinvasive or premalignant changes are called *cervical intraepithelial neoplasia* (CIN)

   ❏ *Classified into three categories (CIN I, II, III) to demonstrate progression of disease and whether disease is considered invasive or malignant*

   CIN I = mild dysplasia

   CIN II = moderate dysplasia

   CIN III = severe dysplasia or CIS

   ❏ *CIN lesions can regress, persist, or become invasive*

❏ *CIN III is more likely to progress than CIN I or II. There is no way to predict which will progress*

5. *Invasive disease* is **malignant disease that extends beyond basement membrane**

❏ *Cervical cancer spreads by three routes*

☐ *Direct extension:* Throughout entire cervix, into parametrium, uterus, bladder, and rectum

☐ *Lymphatics:* Parametrial, paracervical, obturator, hypogastric, external iliac, and sacral nodes

☐ *Hematogenous:* Venous plexus, paracervical veins

☐ *Distant sites:* Lung, liver, bone, mediastinal and supraclavicular nodes

Approaches to Care

■ Assessment

1. Clinical manifestations

❏ *In preinvasive and early stages, asymptomatic except for watery vaginal discharge*

❏ *Later disease symptoms are*
☐ Postcoital bleeding
☐ Intermenstrual bleeding
☐ Heavy menstrual flow
☐ Symptoms related to anemia
☐ Foul-smelling vaginal discharge
☐ Pain in pelvis, hypogastrium, flank, leg
☐ Urinary or rectal symptoms

❏ *End-stage disease*
  ☐ Edema of lower extremities
  ☐ Massive vaginal hemorrhage
  ☐ Renal failure

2. Diagnostic measures

❏ *Pap smear*
  ☐ Most effective tool for assessing and diagnosing cervical cancer
  ☐ Recommended annually for all sexually active women or those over 18 years of age
  ☐ Frequency of smear may be altered by individual's physician

❏ *If smear shows CIN, then*
  ☐ Colposcopy
  ☐ Biopsy
  ☐ Possibly treatment

❏ *Staging is based on clinical findings*
  ☐ Initial staging is best prognostic indicator
  ☐ Five-year survival rates are

    Stage I: 80.5%

    Stage II: 59%

    Stage III: 33%

    Stage IV: 7%

❏ *Clinical work-up for cervical cancer includes*
  ☐ Cervical biopsies
  ☐ Endocervical curettage
  ☐ Cystoscopy

   ☐ Proctosigmoidoscopy

   ☐ Metastatic work-up: Chest x-ray, intravenous pyelogram, barium enema, hematologic profile, liver scan, CT or MRI, node biopsies

■ Interventions

1. **Accurate evaluation of extent of disease is critical**

2. **Treatment for CIN varies greatly from that for invasive disease**

3. **CIN treatment selection**

   ❏ *Is based on extent of disease*

   ❏ *Is based on woman's desire to preserve reproductive function*

   ❏ *Can include*

      ☐ Cervical biopsy

      ☐ Electrocautery

      ☐ Cryosurgery
- Most used method
- Painless
- Low morbidity
- Outpatient setting
- Patients experience watery discharge for 2 to 4 weeks

      ☐ Laser surgery
- 80% to 90% of CIN can be eradicated
- Less disease-free tissue removed
- Slight discomfort
- Little vaginal discharge
- Heals in 2 to 3 weeks

- □ Electrosurgery
  - Increasingly popular
  - Loop electrosurgical excision procedure
  - One outpatient visit
  - Minimal tissue ablation
  - Slight discharge
- □ Cone biopsy
  - Removes cone-shaped piece of tissue from endocervix and exocervix
  - General anesthesia
  - Outpatient procedure
  - Diagnostic or therapeutic
  - Potential hemorrhage or perforation
  - Delayed complications include

    Bleeding

    Cervical stenosis

    Infertility

    Increased chances of preterm delivery

    Complications relate to amount of endocervix removed
- □ Hysterectomy
  - May be used for treatment of post-childbearing women

4. Invasive disease treatment

- ❑ *Based on woman's age, medical condition, and extent of disease*
- ❑ *Either surgery or radiotherapy can be used with equal efficacy for early-stage disease*
- ❑ *In general, stages IIb to IV are initially treated with radiotherapy*

❏ *Treatment selection is related to stage of disease*

☐ Stage Ia (microinvasive)

- Hysterectomy: Abdominal or vaginal

- Conization for patients who are poor surgical risks

☐ Stages Ib and IIa

- Treatment selection is controversial, related to preserving ovarian function

- Radical abdominal hysterectomy and pelvic lymphadenectomy: Ovarian function preserved; vagina more pliable than with radiation; shorter treatment time

- External beam radiotherapy to whole pelvis (5000–8000 cGy) with one or two intracavitary insertions; outpatient care

☐ Stages IIb, III, and IV

- Pretreatment staging laparotomy is controversial; can identify candidates for specific therapies, but is plagued by complications and minimal improvement in survival

- High doses of external beam radiation with parametrial boosts: 5500 to 6000 cGy over 5 to 6 weeks; interstitial implants to supplement

- Intracavitary radiation

- Pelvic exenteration

  Used only in selected group of patients with centralized disease not adherent to pelvic side walls or involving nodes

Complications include

Vaginal stenosis	Cystitis
Fistula	Hemorrhage
Stricture	Abscess

- ☐ Recurrent or persistent disease
  - About 35% of women have recurrent or persistent disease
  - Post-treatment follow-up is critical, though recurrence is difficult to detect
  - Most recurrences occur within 2 years
  - Seventy-five percent of recurrences are local
  - Twenty-five percent of recurrences are distant sites
  - Signs include

    Unexplained weight loss

    Leg edema

    Pain in pelvis or thigh

    Serosanguinous vaginal discharge

    Cough, hemoptysis

  - Triad of weight loss, leg edema, and pelvic pain leads to grim outlook
  - Aim of treatment is palliation
  - Survival averages 6 to 10 months
- ☐ Treatment for recurrent disease is
  - Surgery

    Pelvic exenteration for central recurrence

    Psychosexual and social rehabilitation needed

Postoperative problems include

Embolism

Pulmonary edema

Cerebrovascular accident

Sepsis

Bowel obstruction

Myocardial infarction

- Chemotherapy

  Complicated by decreased pelvic vascular perfusion, limited bone marrow reserve, and poor renal function

  Response rates range from 10% to 40%

  No long-term benefit

  Response rates higher in patients with no prior chemotherapy or radiation

  Cisplatin has greatest single-agent activity

  Other agents include dibromoducitol, ifosfamide, carboplatin

  Combination agents are not more effective

  Pelvic intra-arterial infusions have been tried

  Can be used as radiosensitizer, particularly hydroxyurea or cisplatin

- Radiotherapy

  May be used to treat metastatic disease outside initial radiation field

  Selectively used within previous fields

■ **Nursing management issues are detailed in Chapter 58**

Suggested Readings

1. Walczak J, Klemm PR: Gynecologic cancers. In Groenwald SL, Frogge MH, Goodman M, Yarbro CH (eds.): *Cancer Nursing: Principles and Practice* (3rd ed.). Boston: Jones and Bartlett, 1993, pp. 1084–1099.

2. Meanwell CA: The epidemiology and etiology of cervical cancer. In Blackwell GRP, Jordan JA, and Shingleton HM (eds.): *Textbook of Gynecologic Oncology*. Philadelphia: WB Saunders, 1991, pp. 250–264.

3. Hatch K, Helm CW: Cancer of the cervix: Surgical treatment. In Blackwell GRP, Jordan JA, and Shingleton HM (eds.): *Textbook of Gynecologic Oncology*. Philadelphia: WB Saunders, 1991, pp. 265–280.

4. Greer BE, Berek JS (eds.): *Gynecologic Oncology: Treatment Rationale and Techniques*. New York: Elsevier, 1991.

5. Rose PG, Watkins E, Amyot K, et al: A randomized comparison of hydroxyurea versus hydroxyurea, 5-FU infusion, and bolus cisplatin versus weekly cisplatin as adjunct to radiation therapy in patients with stage IIb, III, IVa carcinoma of the cervix and negative paraortic nodes. Philadelphia: Gynecology Oncology Group, 1992.

▪ 41 ▪

Colon, Rectal, and Anal Cancers

Overview

■ Significant problem in U.S.

■ Incidence rate

1. Fifteen percent of all malignancies

2. There are an estimated 152,000 new cases each year: 109,000 are colon cancer and 43,000 are rectal cancer

3. There are 57,000 deaths each year due to colorectal cancer

■ Occurrence rate

1. Increases after age 40

2. Decreases after age 75

■ Mean age at diagnosis is 63 years

■ Male/female distribution is equal

■ **Native Americans have significantly lower incidence than white Americans**

■ **Africa and Japan have lower incidence than U.S.**

■ **Risk factors**

1. **Dietary factors appear to have dominant role**

   ❏ *Dietary fat and protein increase risk of colon cancer*

   ❏ *High-fiber diets may increase stool transit time and reduce potential of carcinogenic activity*

   ❏ *Fecal bacteria, viruses, and parasites may induce carcinogenic changes*

   ❏ *Calcium may be protective agent and decrease risk*

   ❏ *Chemoprotective agents include ascorbic acid, cruciferous foods*

2. **Predisposing conditions**

   ❏ *Familial adenomatous polyposis*

   ❏ *Gardner's, Oldfield's, Turcot, Peutz-Jeghers syndromes*

   ❏ *Family history of colorectal cancer*

   ❏ *Hereditary adenocarcinomatosis syndrome*

   ❏ *Inflammatory diseases*
      □ Ulcerative colitis
      □ Crohn's disease

■ **Adenocarcinoma is major histologic type**

■ **Anal cancer is rare**

1. **Associated with viruses**

2. **Squamous cell is most common (63%)**

3. **Slow growing; may appear as fistula, hemorrhoid, fissure**

■ **Progression of disease does not relate to symptoms**

■ **Five-year disease-free rates in Dukes' classification system are**

Dukes' A = 67% to 81%

Dukes' B = 51% to 64%

Dukes' C = 32% to 44%

■ **Lymph node involvement occurs in 50% of cases**

■ **Common metastatic sites are liver, lungs, bone, and brain**

Approaches to Care

■ **Assessment**

1. **Clinical manifestations**

   ❏ *Relate to location of tumor*

   ❏ *Many are asymptomatic early in disease*

❏ *Lesions on right side of colon can become large prior to symptoms*
  ☐ Pain that is crampy or pressure-like
  ☐ Occult blood in stool
  ☐ Palpable mass when lesion is large

❏ *Tumors of transverse colon*
  ☐ Occult blood in stool
  ☐ May lead to bowel obstruction and pain

❏ *Tumors of left colon tend to constrict*
  ☐ Sensation of fullness or cramping
  ☐ Changes in bowel habits
  ☐ Bleeding with bright red blood

❏ *Tumors of rectum also constrict*
  ☐ Sense of incomplete evacuation
  ☐ Tenesmus, sense of fullness
  ☐ Stool caliber becomes pencil-like
  ☐ Pain as tumor invades regionally

❏ *Half of patients have lymph node involvement at time of presentation*

2. Diagnostic measures

❏ *Physical examination is focused on*
  ☐ Specific gastrointestinal symptoms
  ☐ Prior medical and family risk factors
  ☐ Palpation for masses
  ☐ Digital examination of rectal area
  ☐ Vaginal examination for fistulas

❏ *Diagnostic studies*
  ☐ Endoscopic examination
  ☐ Barium enema
  ☐ Fecal occult blood testing
  ☐ Carcinoembryonic antigen (CEA) levels

- ☐ CA 19–9 assay

- ☐ Metastatic work-up: abdominal films and scans, liver function studies

❏ *Classification and staging by Dukes' or tumor-node-metastases (TNM) system; both are widely accepted*

■ Interventions

1. Surgery is treatment of choice

❏ *Extent of resection is defined by*
- ☐ Tumor location
- ☐ Blood supply
- ☐ Lymph node patterns in involved region

❏ *Colon cancer common procedures*
- ☐ Right hemicolectomy for tumors of appendix, cecum, ascending colon, and hepatic flexure

- ☐ Transverse colectomy for tumors in that portion of bowel

- ☐ Left hemicolectomy or partial colectomy when splenic flexure and descending colon are involved

- ☐ Partial colectomy is preferred for tumors of distal transverse colon

- ☐ Sigmoid colectomy with remaining colon anastomosed to upper rectum is preferred for sigmoid lesions

- ☐ Subtotal or total colectomy involves removal of most of or entire colon
  - ▪ Nutritional and skin care problems are significant
  - ▪ Reserved for those with large tumors and high probability for cure

- □ Rectal cancer procedures are more specific to region
  - Procedures aimed at sphincter-saving resections are

    Low anterior resection for tumors of distal sigmoid and upper rectum

    Abdominal perineal resection for lesions adjacent to sphincter

    Associated with high morbidity

    Requires extensive adaptation to permanent colostomy

    Requires temporary perineal wound for drainage

    Associated with sexual dysfunction from nerve severance

- □ Anal cancer procedures are selected on tumor-specific criteria of location and stage
  - Small lesions may be treated with local excision, although locoregional recurrence is possible
  - Standard therapy has been abdominoperineal resection
  - Radiation is successful alternative therapy

2. Radiation therapy

❏ *Used as adjuvant therapy to prevent local recurrences*

❏ *Preoperative radiation can*
  - Improve resectability
  - Reduce viability of malignant cells
  - Lessen chance of local recurrence

❏ *Combined preoperative and postoperative radiation*
  ☐ Referred to as "sandwich technique"
  ☐ Used to decrease potential for tumor dissemination
  ☐ Potential for complication of repopulation by residual cells if postoperative therapy is delayed because of slow wound healing
  ☐ Postoperative radiotherapy
    ■ Used for those who are considered at high risk for local recurrence
    ■ Distant metastases still potential problem
  ☐ Palliative radiation
    ■ Effective in treating symptoms of advanced cancer
    ■ Pain and bleeding can be controlled
  ☐ Endocavitary radiation used as local treatment for rectal cancer
  ☐ Intraoperative radiation used for locally advanced, recurrent, or inoperable rectal cancer
  ☐ Brachytherapy implants of radioactive seeds or afterloading techniques used for pelvic recurrence
  ☐ Hyperthermia used as adjunct therapy to radiation and chemotherapy
  ☐ Laser therapy used for inoperable tumors of rectum or descending colon

3. Chemotherapy
  ❏ *Colorectal cancer appears to be extremely resistant to chemotherapy*

❏ *5-Fluorouracil (5-FU) is most researched and used single agent*

❏ *Continuous infusions of 5-FU for protracted periods improve response rates*

❏ *Levamisole has been added to many 5-FU regimens*
  ❏ Immunorestorative activity seems to enhance effects of 5-FU

❏ *Other single and combination agent regimens have been tried, but with limited success*

❏ *Anal cancer most effectively treated with combination radiation and chemotherapy*

4. Alternative therapies

❏ *Biologic response modifiers being investigated*

❏ *Alpha-interferon and interleukin-2 have demonstrated varying degrees of activity and response*

Suggested Readings

1. Hampton B: Gastrointestinal cancer: Colon, rectum, and anus. In Groenwald SL, Frogge MH, Goodman M, Yarbro CH (eds.): *Cancer Nursing: Principles and Practice* (3rd ed.). Boston: Jones and Bartlett, 1993, pp. 1044–1064.

2. Ahlgren JD, Macdonald JS (eds.): *Gastrointestinal Oncology*. Philadelphia: Lippincott, 1992, pp. 243–395.

3. Fitzsimmons ML: Hereditary colorectal cancers. *Semin Oncol Nurs* 8:252–257, 1992.

▪ 42 ▪
Endocrine Cancers

Overview

■ **Most common endocrine malignancies are**

1. Thyroid cancer

❏ *Rare; accounts for approximately 1% of total cancers and approximately 0.2% of cancer deaths*

❏ *Women have more than 2 times risk of developing thyroid cancer*

❏ *Most cases occur between ages of 25 and 65 years*

❏ *Higher incidence in adults who received head and neck irradiation during childhood or adolescence*

❏ *Medullary thyroid cancer associated with genetically transmitted multiple endocrine neoplasia (MEN) syndrome*

❏ *Types*
  ☐ Papillary carcinoma
    ▪ Indolent
    ▪ Survival measured in decades, even in patients with metastases
    ▪ Cervical lymph node involvement usually occurs early in disease
    ▪ Metastasis occurs to lungs and, less frequently, to bone
    ▪ Occurs in all age groups
    ▪ Biologic behavior and prognosis vary by age; tumors in patients older than 40 years are more aggressive and rapidly growing
    ▪ Death usually caused by recurrent or uncontrolled local disease, even with distant metastases
  ☐ Follicular carcinoma
    ▪ Tends to be more locally invasive than papillary form
    ▪ Average age at diagnosis is 45 to 50 years
    ▪ Cervical lymph node involvement common
    ▪ Bone metastases more frequent
    ▪ May retain ability to produce T3 and T4 thyroid hormones, causing hyperthyroidism
    ▪ Poorer prognosis with tumors that have capsular or vascular invasion
    ▪ Death usually caused by growth of local recurrences

- ☐ Medullary carcinoma
  - Approximately 20% of cases occur as part of genetically transmitted MEN syndrome
  - Especially virulent
  - Incidence equal in both sexes
  - Diagnosis usually made at 45 to 50 years of age
  - Lymph node involvement is present in approximately 50% of cases; metastasis occurs later in lung, bone, and liver
- ☐ Anaplastic carcinoma
  - Generally rapidly growing and lethal, with death occurring within months of diagnosis
  - Females affected more often than males
  - Average age at diagnosis is 65 years
  - Local invasion is common
  - Metastasizes to lung

2. Pituitary tumors

- ❏ *Rare*
- ❏ *Occur primarily in middle-aged and older adults*
- ❏ *Many adenomas are well-differentiated, slow-growing, and confined, retaining their hormone-producing capabilities; however, tumor cells do not respond to normal regulatory mechanisms of body, producing hormones regardless of feedback from target organs*
- ❏ *Others are more aggressive, invading adjacent tissue and compressing vital structures*

3. Adrenal tumors

❏ *Rare*

❏ *Incidence same for men and women*

❏ *In 60% to 70% of patients, functional tumors produce excessive amounts of corticosteroids*

❏ *Types*
   ☐ Adrenocortical carcinomas
      ■ Aggressive malignancies; most patients have locally advanced or metastatic disease on diagnosis
      ■ Most common sites of metastases are lung, liver, and lymph nodes
      ■ Local tumor extension involves kidneys, liver, vena cava, pancreas, and diaphragm
   ☐ Pheochromocytomas
      ■ Rare, catecholamine-secreting benign or malignant tumors
      ■ Occasionally associated with other endocrine tumors as part of MEN syndrome
      ■ Genetic predisposition exists

4. Parathyroid tumors

❏ *Rare; account for 1% to 4% of all cases of primary hyperparathyroidism*

❏ *Increased risk for those with previous head and neck irradiation, especially in childhood*

❏ *Most are biologically functional and cause clinical effects of hypercalcemia because of hypersecretion of parathyroid hormone*

❏ *Prolonged survival has been seen, even in patients with metastatic disease*

Approaches to Patient Care

■ Thyroid cancers

1. Assessment

❑ *Clinical manifestations*

  ☐ Most commonly present asymptomatically with thyroid mass and cervical adenopathy

  ☐ Patients may have sensation of tightness or fullness in neck, which may progress to dyspnea or stridor if trachea is compressed or infiltrated

  ☐ Hoarseness or dysphagia may result from infiltration or destruction of recurrent laryngeal or vagus nerves by malignant cells

  ☐ Pain is uncommon and is usually sign of advanced disease

❑ *Diagnostic evaluation*

  ☐ Patient history includes family history, prior irradiation, and rate of tumor growth

  ☐ Physical examination includes checking thyroid and adjacent neck structures and regional lymph nodes for symmetry and palpating for masses

  ☐ Patients with thyroid nodule should undergo examination of head and neck by laryngoscopy

  ☐ Evaluation of altered hormone secretion

    ■ Symptoms of hyperthyroidism
      Fine tremors
      Lid lag
      Brisk tendon reflexes

Increased appetite and weight loss

Tachycardia

Heat intolerance

Proptosis

Irritability

Muscle weakness

- Symptoms of hypothyroidism

Dry skin	*Slowed speech*
Hair loss	*Bradycardia*
Cold intolerance	*Decreased reflexes*
Weight gain	*Constipation*

☐ Fine-needle aspiration is most widely used technique to evaluate nodular thyroid disease

☐ Radionuclide imaging of thyroid provides information about its functional status

- Normal thyroid tissue concentrates iodine and is labeled "warm," nonfunctioning nodules are "cold," and hyperfunctioning nodules are "hot"

- Test does not distinguish benign from malignant nodules

☐ If thyroid dysfunction is suspected, laboratory tests are obtained, including radioactive iodine uptake, T3 uptake, total T4, free T4, and thyroid-stimulating hormone (TSH)

☐ TSH is suppressed by administration of thyroxine to reduce size of nodules and prevent prolonged TSH stimulation of thyroid

2. Treatment

❏ *Thyroid malignancies are managed aggressively*

❏ *Total thyroidectomy*

  ☐ Results in fewer local recurrences and increases effectiveness of ^{131}I therapy

  ☐ Recommended for those with medullary thyroid cancer because of high incidence of bilateral involvement of thyroid gland

  ☐ May require tracheostomy and gastrostomy, which can be performed at time of initial surgery

  ☐ If nodes are involved, lymph node dissection is indicated

  ☐ Thyroid suppressive treatment is given for several weeks before surgery to induce atrophy of thyroid and reduce vascularity and hemorrhage at time of surgery

  ☐ Postoperative complications

    ▪ Hemorrhage because of high vascularity of gland

      Place patient in semi-Fowler's position

      Assess hourly for bleeding

      Assess for increased pressure at surgical site

      Evaluate patency of suction catheters

      Measure fluids

    ▪ Hypoparathyroidism caused by hypofunctioning parathyroid glands

    ▪ Hypocalcemia

      Monitor serum calcium daily

      Replace calcium as necessary

      Watch for signs including

        Numbness

        Tingling

        Cramps in extremities

Stiffening

Twitching

Positive Chvostek's or Trousseau's sign

- Potential damage to recurrent laryngeal nerve causing temporary or permanent vocal cord paralysis, leading to respiratory obstruction

  Keep tracheostomy set at patient's bedside for first 24 hours after surgery

  Emergency tracheostomy may be required

❏ *Radiotherapy*
  □ ^{131}I for ablation or treatment, or both, after surgical resection
    - Isotope concentrates in functional tumor tissue, facilitating cancer cell death
    - Patient admitted to hospital for 48 hours, after which patient is no longer radioactive
  □ Complications
    - Nausea and vomiting
    - Fatigue
    - Headache
    - Bone marrow suppression
    - Sialadenitis
    - Rarely, pulmonary radiation fibrosis and leukemia
  □ External beam radiation may be useful in palliation of painful bony metastases

❏ *Chemotherapy*
  □ Only doxorubicin has shown any significant antitumor activity

❏ *Follow-up of patients*
- ☐ Long-term follow-up important because of risk of late recurrence
- ☐ Serum thyroglobulin and serial isotope scanning are useful in locating recurrent disease
- ☐ Measurement of basal and stimulated calcitonin levels is useful in locating recurrent medullary thyroid cancer

◼ Pituitary tumors

1. Assessment

❏ *Clinical manifestations*
- ☐ Alterations in hormonal patterns
- ☐ Symptoms of compression
  - ▪ Headache
  - ▪ Visual disturbances
  - ▪ Functional impairment of cranial nerves

❏ *Diagnostic measures*
- ☐ Complete evaluation of endocrine system to help define functional status of tumor
- ☐ High-resolution MRI provides information about tumor margins and tumor's effect on adjacent structures
- ☐ Angiography to evaluate lumen of blood vessels; indicated if there is any concern about aneurysm

2. Treatment

❏ *Surgery*
- ☐ Treatment of choice is complete or subtotal resection followed by postoperative radiation therapy; achieves normalization of hormone levels most rapidly

- For most adenomas, transsphenoidal route is adequate, permitting selective removal of tumor and preservation of normal pituitary tissue

- Complications

  Diabetes insipidus

  Cerebrospinal fluid leak

  Meningitis

- During recovery period, sneezing and nose blowing are contraindicated to minimize pressure on operative site

- Pituitary hormone levels are measured after surgery to assess effectiveness of removal of hypersecreting tumor tissue

❏ *Radiotherapy*

  ☐ Indicated

   - When tumor is not resectable

   - To manage patients with incompletely resected or recurrent tumors

   - For treatment of some patients with persistent hyperfunctioning endocrinopathies

  ☐ Major complication is hypopituitarism

   - Monitor endocrine function continuously

❏ *Pharmacotherapy*

  ☐ Dopamine antagonists or somatostatin analogs may be used to treat hypersecreting pituitary adenomas to reduce hormone levels and shrink tumor

■ Adrenal cortical carcinomas

1. Assessment

❏ *Clinical manifestations*

- ☐ Patients with nonfunctional tumors usually have palpable abdominal mass and may have abdominal or back pain

- ☐ Fever, weight loss, weakness, and lethargy are seen primarily in patients with advanced disease

- ☐ Patients with functional tumors will have excess production of one or more hormones secreted by adrenal cortex
  - Most functional tumors result in Cushing's disease, virilization and feminization syndromes, and hyperaldosteronism

❏ *Diagnostic measures*

- ☐ Functional tumors are detected by immunoassays of hormone precursors and mature hormones

- ☐ CT is used most commonly to localize tumors; it provides information about hepatic, renal, and vena cava involvement

- ☐ MRI can be used to differentiate benign adenomas from adrenocortical carcinomas and pheochromocytomas

2. Treatment

❏ *Surgery is treatment of choice and may be curative for localized disease*

❏ *Glucocorticoid treatment may be needed either temporarily or permanently*

❑ *Drugs used in treatment act either by causing necrosis of adrenal cortex (mitotane) or by blocking corticosteroid secretion (aminoglutethimide); either may be used as adjuvant therapy or for treatment of inoperable disease*

❑ *Chemotherapy has limited activity*

❑ *Radiation therapy does not improve overall survival, but may palliate symptoms of invasive or metastatic cancer*

■ **Pheochromocytomas**

1. **Assessment**

❑ *Clinical manifestations*

☐ Excess production of catecholamines accounts for most of tumor's clinical manifestations

☐ Sustained or paroxysmal diastolic hypertension may be present

☐ Other symptoms

- Headache
- Sweating
- Nausea and vomiting
- Palpitations
- Anxiety

❑ *Diagnostic measures*

☐ Diagnosis confirmed by measuring urinary and circulating catecholamines or their metabolites

☐ CT scan is used to localize tumor

☐ Meta-iodobenzylguanidine (MIBG) scan helps localize tumor

2. Treatment

- ❏ *Surgery is treatment of choice*

- ❏ *Patients are monitored for signs of shock related to abrupt decrease in circulating catecholamines*

▰ Parathyroid tumors

1. Assessment

- ❏ *Clinical manifestions*
  - ☐ Hyperparathyroidism may be seen as elevated calcium level on routine laboratory evaluation or may be found incidentally during work-up for other unrelated symptoms
  - ☐ Bone pain
  - ☐ Urolithiasis
  - ☐ Neuropsychiatric changes
  - ☐ Gastrointestinal symptoms
  - ☐ Palpable neck masses are seen rarely

- ❏ *Diagnostic measures*
  - ☐ Nuclear scanning, CT, and ultrasound are most useful methods to localized parathyroid mass
  - ☐ Approximately one-half of patients with hyperparathyroidism have evidence of bony disease

2. Treatment

- ❏ *Surgery includes en bloc resection of abnormal parathyroid; if nodes are involved, radical neck dissection is done*

- ❏ *Surgery may be used to resect recurrent disease; not curative, but helps control hypercalcemia and disease symptoms*

❏ *Postoperative complications include*
  ▢ Hypoparathyroidism
  ▢ Recurrent laryngeal nerve damage
  ▢ Hemorrhage

❏ *Neither radiation nor chemotherapy have been successful in treating either primary or metastatic disease*

Suggested Readings

1. Donehower MG: Endocrine cancers. In Groenwald SL, Frogge MH, Goodman M, Yarbro CH (eds.): *Cancer Nursing: Principles and Practice* (3rd ed.). Boston: Jones and Bartlett, 1993, pp. 984–1003.

2. Kenady DE, Sloan DA, Schwartz RW: Diagnosis and treatment of thyroid, adrenal and thymic tumors. *Current Opin Oncol* 4:89–98, 1992.

3. Decker RA, Kuehner ME: Adrenocortical carcinoma. *Am Surg* 57:502–513, 1991.

■ 43 ■
Endometrial Cancers

Overview

■ Predominant cancer of female genital tract

■ Mortality rate is low

■ About 31,000 new cases diagnosed in 1993

■ Only approximately 5700 women died of the disease in 1993

■ Over 79% of women are diagnosed when disease is localized

■ Overall good prognosis

■ Survival rates are

1. Stage I: 76%
2. Stage II: 50%

3. Stage III: 30%

4. Stage IV: 9%

■ Primarily disease of postmenopausal women

■ Most women are diagnosed between 50 and 59 years of age

■ Risk factors

1. Obesity (>20 lb overweight)

2. Nulliparity

3. Late menopause (>52 yrs of age)

4. Diabetes

5. Hypertension

6. Infertility

7. Irregular menses

8. History of breast or ovarian cancer

9. Adenomatous hyperplasia

10. Prolonged use of estrogen therapy

■ Ninety percent of tumors are adenocarcinomas

■ Multiple factors affect prognosis

1. Histologic type and differentiation

2. Uterine size

3. Stage of disease

4. Pattern or degree of invasion (especially myometrial)

■ **Metastatic spread is usually to**

1. Pelvic and para-aortic nodes

2. Vagina

3. Peritoneal cavity

4. Omentum

5. Inguinal lymph nodes

6. Lung

7. Liver

8. Bone

9. Brain

Approaches to Care

■ **Assessment**

1. **Clinical manifestations**
   - ❏ *Abnormal vaginal bleeding is hallmark signal*
   - ❏ *Most women with endometrial cancer are postmenopausal*
   - ❏ *Less common symptoms are*
     - ☐ Premenopausal onset of heavy or irregular bleeding
     - ☐ Pyometra
     - ☐ Hematuria
     - ☐ Lumbosacral, hypogastric, or pelvic pain

2. **Diagnostic measures**
   - ❏ *Thorough pelvic examination*
   - ❏ *Endometrial biopsy*

❏ *Chest x-ray*

❏ *Intravenous pyelogram*

❏ *Hematologic profiles*

❏ *Cystoscopy, barium enema, proctoscopy*

■ Interventions

1. Primary treatment is surgical

❏ *Surgical procedures involve*

☐ Bimanual examination

☐ Peritoneal cytology

☐ Inspection and palpation of peritoneal surfaces

☐ Biopsies

☐ Selective pelvic and para-aortic lymphadenectomy

☐ Total abdominal hysterectomy

☐ Bilateral salpingo-oophorectomy

☐ Possible omentectomy

❏ *Adjuvant radiation therapy for early cancer is sometimes used*

☐ If there is positive peritoneal cytology, intraperitoneal radioactive colloidal phosphorous can be helpful

☐ External beam therapy is used for disease localized to pelvis

☐ Whole-pelvis radiation allows treatment of all pelvic tissue

2. Advanced or recurrent disease treatment is difficult

❏ *Vaginal recurrences are treated with surgery or radiotherapy*

❏ *Hormonal therapy or chemotherapy are used for recurrences outside vagina*

  ☐ Hormone therapy

    ▪ Synthetic progestational agents produce 30% to 37% response rates

    ▪ Receptor status greatly affects response

    ▪ If both estrogen and progesterone receptors are positive, response rate is 77%

    ▪ Megestrol acetate and medroxyprogesterone are most commonly used

  ☐ Chemotherapy

    ▪ Few agents are effective

    ▪ Doxorubicin every 3 weeks is common

    ▪ High-dose cisplatin (100 mg/m^2) is used as first-line therapy, with little effect on refractory disease

■ Information needs related to endometrial cancer

1. Estrogen replacement therapy (ERT)

❏ *Indications for use*

  ☐ Vaginal atrophy with infection or sexual dysfunction

  ☐ Loss of pelvic support with incontinence

  ☐ Postmenopausal osteoporosis

  ☐ Perimenopausal emotional lability

  ☐ Early surgical or radiation castration

  ☐ Vasomotor instability

  ☐ Lowered morbidity and mortality for cardiovascular disease

❑ *Estrogen cycled with progesterone*

❑ *Annual pelvic exam, histologic sampling of endometrium, and mammogram*

❑ *Seek medical attention if any abnormal vaginal bleeding occurs including postmenopausal bleeding*

2. Breast self-examination (BSE)

❑ *Importance of BSE in conjunction with ERT*

❑ *Technique for performing BSE and demonstration of skill*

3. Diet and weight control

❑ *Low-fat, calcium-rich diet*
❑ *Maintain weight within normal range*
❑ *Weight-bearing exercises to decrease bone loss*

4. Abnormal vaginal bleeding

❑ *Seek medical attention for new onset of abnormal bleeding*

❑ *Evaluation includes pelvic examination and endometrial biopsy*

5. Sexual role functioning

❑ *Dispel myths related to perceived loss of femininity due to surgery*

❑ *Help redefine self in terms other than reproduction*

6. Sexual functioning

❑ *Complete sexual assessment*

❏ *Alteration in sexual response secondary to hysterectomy*
  ☐ Cervix contributes to but is not essential for orgasm
  ☐ Uterus elevates during excitement phase and contracts rhythmically during orgasm

❏ *Alteration in sexual functioning secondary to radiation*
  ☐ Vaginal dryness and stenosis may result in patient who is not sexually active, unless vaginal dilators and lubricants are employed
  ☐ Use of water-soluble lubricants during intercourse. Use of nonhormonal moisturizers three times per week

Suggested Readings

1. Walczak JR, Klemm PR: Gynecologic cancers. In Groenwald SL, Frogge MH, Goodman M, Yarbro CH (eds.): *Cancer Nursing: Principles and Practice* (3rd ed.). Boston: Jones and Bartlett, 1993, pp. 1065–1072.

2. DiSaia PJ, Creasman WT: *Clinical Gynecologic Oncology.* St. Louis: Mosby, 1989.

3. Hubbard JL, Holcombe JK: Cancer of the endometrium. *Semin Oncol Nurs* 6:206–213, 1990.

4. Hacker NF: Uterine cancer. In Berek JS, Hacker NF (eds.): *Practical Gynecologic Oncology.* Baltimore: Williams & Wilkins, 1989, pp. 285–326.

■ 44 ■
Esophageal Tumors

Overview

- Grow rapidly, metastasize early, and are diagnosed late

- Survival rates are poor

- Uncommon in U.S.

- Represent 1% of all cancer cases and 2% of cancer deaths

- Only 7% of those affected will be alive 5 years after diagnosis

- More common among men than women

- African American males have highest incidence

- Average age of onset is 62 years

■ Risk factors include

1. Heavy alcohol intake
2. Poor nutrition
3. Anemia
4. Untreated achalasia
5. Plummer-Vinson syndrome
6. Heavy tobacco use
7. Cirrhosis
8. Poor oral hygiene
9. Chronic irritation
10. Barrett's syndrome

■ Histologic types

1. Squamous cell carcinoma: Dominant type
2. Adenocarcinoma

■ Metastasis occurs by

1. Continuous extension
2. Lymphatic spread
3. Hematologic spread

Approaches to Care

■ Assessment

1. Clinical manifestations

❑ *Many people mistakenly attribute signs and symptoms to disorders of digestion that commonly affect older persons*

❑ *Early symptoms may be nonspecific and of little concern*

❑ *Definitive symptoms may be present for only weeks or months and disease may be well advanced*

❑ *Initial symptoms include pressure, fullness, indigestion, substernal distress*

❑ *Dysphagia is the classic symptom in 90% of cases*

❑ *Dysphagia is progressive and patient will attempt to modify food intake and mastication to accommodate progressive obstruction*

❑ *Pain on swallowing occurs in 50% of cases*

❑ *Weight loss is dramatic, sometimes 10% to 20% of body weight*

2. Diagnostic measures

❑ *Routine x-ray films and double-barium contrast studies*

❑ *CT scan for staging*

❑ *Endoscopy and biopsy*

❏ *Cytologic studies for tissue diagnosis*

❏ *Endoscopic ultrasound for staging*

■ Treatment

1. Pretreatment preparation includes

❏ *Intensive nutritional therapy*
❏ *Pulmonary hygiene*
❏ *Chest physiotherapy*
❏ *Control of secretions*

2. Surgery, radiation, and chemotherapy are options; a combination of the three appear to offer best alternative

❏ *Radiotherapy*

☐ Can result in rapid relief of obstruction

☐ Excellent modality for combination therapy

☐ Alternative for palliation of advanced disease

☐ Complications of radiotherapy

- Swallowing difficulties
- Skin reactions
- Esophageal fistula
- Stricture
- Radiation pneumonitis

❏ *Preoperative radiotherapy can*

☐ Reduce tumor bulk
☐ Improve surgical resectability
☐ Improve swallowing and nutritional status

❏ *Postoperative radiotherapy can*

☐ Eradicate residual tumor cells in surgical site
☐ Be used for local control

- ❏ *Intracavitary radiation*
  - ☐ Implants placed via endoscope
  - ☐ Provide therapeutic boost dose to local area

- ❏ *Surgery*
  - ☐ Employed selectively at all three levels of esophagus
  - ☐ Goal may be to cure or palliate
  - ☐ Curative intent
    - ▪ Eradicate tumor
    - ▪ Reestablish esophageal continuity
    - ▪ Stage I and II tumors without evidence of local or distant metastases are eligible
  - ☐ Palliative intent
    - ▪ Maintain esophageal patency
    - ▪ Improve quality of life
  - ☐ Surgical approaches
    - ▪ Left transthoracic approach for cancers of lower third of esophagus
    - ▪ Right thoracotomy with laparotomy for cancers of upper and middle third of esophagus
    - ▪ Transhiatal esophagectomy for cancer at all three levels
    - ▪ En bloc resection for tumors of lower esophagus and cardia. If cure is possible, resection is extended
    - ▪ Reconstruction of esophageal continuity can be achieved by

      Elevating stomach to create esophagogastrectomy

Interposing segment of colon

Elevating gastric tube created from stomach to reconstruct lumen

- Special considerations necessary for cervical esophagus because of difficulties imposed by tumor location including

  Radical neck dissection

  Partial cervical esophagectomy

  Reconstruction done with initial procedure or as second-stage procedure

❑ *Postoperative care*

  ☐ Potential complications are

  - Fistula
  - Atelectasis
  - Adult respiratory distress syndrome
  - Anastomotic leak
  - Pneumonia
  - Pulmonary edema

❑ *Important nursing measures are*

  ☐ Give preoperative antibiotic regimen

  ☐ Aggressive respiratory care

  ☐ Tracheal intubation care

  ☐ Chest physiotherapy

  ☐ Chest tube care

  ☐ Tracheobronchial hygiene

  ☐ Prevent fluid overload

  ☐ Prevent infection

  ☐ Antibiotic therapy

  ☐ Meticulous suture line care

  ☐ Monitor drainage, output

  ☐ Reduce anastomosis tension

- □ Maintain patent gastrointestinal tubes
- □ Help patient to maintain body alignment
- □ Detect fistulas
- □ Prevent reflux aspiration
- □ Elevate head of bed
- □ Encourage patient not to consume snacks or liquid after evening meal
- □ Encourage patient to eat small amounts of food more often
- □ Encourage patient to avoid bending from waist
- □ Encourage patient to avoid heavy lifting
- □ Control odor (with colon interposition)
  - ▪ Help patient to maintain meticulous oral hygiene
  - ▪ Encourage patient to avoid gas-producing foods
  - ▪ Encourage use of mint candies
  - ▪ Suggest use of charcoal carbonate tablets

❏ *Chemotherapy*
  - □ Agents currently used are
    - ▪ Cisplatin
    - ▪ Mitomycin-C
    - ▪ Doxorubicin
    - ▪ Vindesine
    - ▪ 5-fluorouracil
    - ▪ Mitoguazone
    - ▪ Bleomycin
  - □ Sequenced chemotherapy in multimodal approach offers promise
  - □ Preoperative chemoradiation therapy
    - ▪ Delivers local and systemic therapy simultaneously
    - ▪ Severe mucositis and myelosuppression are limiting toxicities

❏ *Palliative therapy*

  ☐ Radiotherapy of 3000 to 5000 cGy decreases tumor size and bleeding

  ☐ Laser therapy alleviates esophageal obstruction and severe dysphagia

  ☐ Resection or bypass relieves severe symptoms or reduces tumor bulk

  ☐ Synthetic endoesophageal prosthetic tubes create open passage for swallowing

    ▪ Care of person with endoprosthesis includes

      Educating patient

      Preventing of reflux up tube

      Elevating head of bed

      Helping patient take all meals in upright position

      Helping patient to eat smaller amounts of food more often

      Helping patient to dislodge trapped food with nasogastric tube

      Helping patient to drink half glass of water or carbonated beverage at end of meal to clear tube

Suggested Readings

1. Frogge MH: Gastrointestinal cancer: Esophagus, stomach, liver, and pancreas. In Groenwald SL, Frogge MH, Goodman M, Yarbro CH (eds.): *Cancer Nursing: Principles and Practice* (3rd ed.). Boston: Jones and Bartlett, 1993, pp. 1004–1017.

2. Klumpp TR, Macdonald JS: Esophageal cancer: Epidemiology and pathology. In Ahlgren JD, Macdonald JS (eds.): *Gastrointestinal Oncology.* Philadelphia: Lippincott, 1992, pp. 71–80.

3. Ellis FH: Esophageal carcinoma. In Steele G, Cady B (eds.): *General Surgical Oncology.* Philadelphia: WB Saunders, 1992, pp. 87–106.

4. Davydov MI, Akhvlediani GG, Stilidi IS, et al: Surgical aspects in the treatment of esophageal cancer. *Semin Surg Oncol* 8:4–8, 1992.

■ 45 ■
Head and Neck Malignancies

Overview

■ Represent 5% of total newly diagnosed cancers in U.S.

■ Incidence is 40% in cancer of oral cavity, 25% in laryngeal cancer, 17% in cancers of oropharynx and hypopharynx, 7% in cancers of major salivary glands, and 13% in remaining sites

■ Male to female incidence ratio is 3:1

■ Incidence increases with age

■ Usually locally aggressive; spread first to sites within head and neck

■ Risk factors

1. Use of tobacco, including cigarettes, smokeless tobacco, pipes, cigars

2. Use of alcohol; there may also be synergism between alcohol and tobacco

3. Exposure to dust from wood, metal, leather, or textiles

4. Poor oral hygiene; chronic irritation from loose-fitting dentures

5. Epstein-Barr virus (EBV)

6. Genetic predisposition

7. Nutritional deficiencies such as Plummer-Vinson syndrome

8. Vitamin A deficiency

■ Approximately 95% are squamous cell in origin

■ Most invade locally, deep into underlying structures, and along tissue planes; invasion into bone usually occurs late in disease

■ Important factor in determining prognosis is presence or absence of histologically proved lymph node metastasis

■ Approximately 30% of individuals have second primary tumor; greatest risk of second primary tumor occurs within first 3-year period after treatment for primary cancer

■ Types of head and neck cancers

1. Carcinoma of nasal cavity and paranasal sinuses

❑ *Maxillary sinus most commonly affected site*

❑ *Affects individuals older than age 40; affects men twice as often as women*

❑ *Risk factors: Exposure to*
   ☐ Leather or nickel plating or work in furniture manufacturing
   ☐ Chromate compounds
   ☐ Hydrocarbons
   ☐ Nitrosamines
   ☐ Mustard gas
   ☐ Isopropyl alcohol
   ☐ Petroleum
   ☐ Dioxane

2. Carcinoma of nasopharynx

❑ *Incidence ratio of males to females is 3:1*

❑ *Appears to be viral association with EBV*

❑ *Genetic predisposition may exist in individuals from southern China; related to size of nasal cavity and ingestion of salted fish*

3. Carcinoma of oral cavity

❑ *Cure rates increase dramatically if disease is diagnosed early when tumor is small*

❑ *Risk factors*
   ☐ Smoking
   ☐ Alcohol abuse

- ☐ Systemic syphilis
- ☐ Poor oral hygiene
- ☐ Poorly fitting dentures or dental appliances
- ☐ Chewing betel nuts

❏ *Approximately 37% of individuals develop multiple primary cancers concurrently or subsequently*

❏ *Not age- or sex-specific*

4. Carcinoma of hypopharynx

❏ *Incidence ratio of males to females is 2:1*

❏ *Most commonly affected sites are*
- ☐ Pyriform sinus (70%)
- ☐ Postcricoid (15%)
- ☐ Posterolateral wall (15%)

❏ *Contributing causes include*
- ☐ Excessive smoking
- ☐ Drinking alcohol
- ☐ Plummer-Vinson syndrome

5. Carcinoma of larynx

❏ *Approximately 80% occur in persons older than 50 years*

❏ *Risk factors*
- ☐ Use of tobacco and alcohol
- ☐ Previous exposure to ionizing radiation

❏ *Multiple primary tumors occur in 5% to 10% of patients*

❏ *Divided into three types according to distinct anatomic areas*
  ☐ *Glottic carcinoma:* Located in space between true cords, including vocal folds and anterior and posterior glottis
  ☐ *Supraglottic carcinoma:* Located in area and structures above glottis, including epiglottis, aryepiglottic folds, arytenoids, and ventricular bands (*false cords*)
  ☐ *Subglottic carcinoma:* Located in area and structures below glottis

Approaches to Patient Care

■ Carcinoma of nasal cavity and paranasal sinuses

1. Assessment

❏ *Clinical manifestations*
  ☐ Symptoms of early disease mimic chronic sinusitis; later symptoms include
■ Stuffy nose	■ Epistaxis
■ Sinus headache	■ Cheek hypesthesia
■ Dull facial pain	■ Trismus
■ Rhinorrhea	■ Loose teeth

❏ *Diagnostic measures*
  ☐ Physical findings may include
    ■ Diplopia
    ■ Proptosis
    ■ Submucosal palatal mass
    ■ Maxillary fullness
    ■ Cranial nerve deficit

- ☐ Cervical adenopathy is unfavorable finding that occurs in 10% of patients at diagnosis

2. Treatment

- ❏ *Early disease may be treated with either radiation or surgery; more advanced disease is usually treated with combination of radiation, surgery, and sometimes chemotherapy*

- ❏ *Surgery*
  - ☐ Maxillectomy is treatment of choice for tumors in maxillary sinus; combination of radical maxillectomy and orbital exenteration may be performed if there is extensive disease with invasion into floor of orbit
    - Before surgery impression is made of hard and soft palate
    - Obturator is made and placed at time of surgery to restore nasal continuity, allow patient to eat and speak immediately after surgery, and protect wound from irritation and debris
    - Obturator remains in place for 5 days; it is then removed and replaced with more permanent obturator
      - *Teach patient to remove obturator after each meal, irrigate it with alkaline-based fluid, and remove any crusting over defect*
      - *Do not remove obturator for long periods of time, as atrophy can occur*
      - *Monitor patients receiving chemotherapy or radiation therapy, or both, for mucositis*
  - ☐ Cranial base surgery
    - Used to resect tumors that involve or have extended to skull base

- Complications

    *Loss of vision if orbital exenteration is
    necessary*

    Temporary facial paralysis

    Loss of feeling in middle or lower face

    Loss of smell if olfactory nerves are transected

❑ *Local recurrence develops in 30% to 40% of
patients with nasal and paranasal cavity
cancer and in 60% of patients with maxillary
sinus cancer*

■ Carcinoma of nasopharynx

1. Assessment

❑ *Clinical manifestations*

  □ First indicator may be presence of enlarged
  node in neck

  □ Nasal obstruction (with or without epistaxis)

  □ Hearing impairment and tinnitus secondary
  to eustachian tube obstruction

  □ Otitis media

  □ Late in disease, headache and facial pain may
  signify bony erosion and pressure on fifth
  cranial nerve

  □ Tumor invasion through base of skull results
  in cranial nerve involvement, causing cranial
  nerve abnormalities

❑ *Diagnostic measures*

  □ Physical examination with head mirror,
  tongue depressor, and laryngeal mirror

  □ Palpate neck nodes thoroughly

□ CT scans and other radiographic tools such as angiography help to determine spread of disease and potential collateralization in cerebrovascular tree

2. Treatment

❏ *Radiotherapy is primary treatment*

❏ *Chemotherapy may be given in conjunction with radiation to potentiate effects of radiation*

■ Carcinoma of oral cavity

1. Assessment

❏ *Many people deny symptoms and do not seek medical help until lesion is large and painful*

❏ *Referred pain to ear or jaw can indicate ulceration or pressure on adjacent nerves*

❏ *Individual may have difficulty chewing and swallowing as lesion progresses*

2. Treatment

❏ *Determined by tumor size*

❏ *In early-stage lesions, surgery or radiation alone have comparable cure rates; choice of treatment depends on*
   □ Functional and cosmetic results required
   □ Patient's general health
   □ Patient's preference

❏ *Chemotherapy used as adjuvant therapy; also plays role in palliation of symptoms in patients whose disease is not curable*

❑ *In oral cavity, surgical resection often involves neck dissection in continuity with tumor and regional lymph nodes*

❑ *Speaking and swallowing can be greatly affected depending on location of tumor*

❑ *Laser therapy is very precise and helps decrease possibility of tumor spread by sealing lymphatics as tissue is removed*

■ Carcinoma of hypopharynx

1. Assessment

❑ *Clinical manifestations*

☐ Presenting symptoms include odynophagia, referred otalgia (usually unilateral), and dysphagia

☐ Weight loss as result of difficulty swallowing food

☐ Hoarseness or aspiration with more advanced disease

❑ *Diagnostic measures*

☐ Physical examination of pharyngeal wall and pyriform sinus is with laryngeal mirror and tongue depressor

☐ Diagnostic studies include CT, direct laryngoscopy, and biopsy

☐ Cervical esophageal extension should be suspected if any of following are found

■ Laryngeal tumor involvement

■ Tumor invasion and mucosal involvement of posterior wall of pharynx

■ Pooling of saliva in or around pyriform sinus and pharynx

2. Treatment

❏ *Most patients have advanced disease at first presentation*

❏ *Surgery may be extensive and necessitate intricate reconstruction using skin and muscle flaps to facilitate closure*

❏ *Swallowing is often problem after surgery because resection of pharyngeal constrictors interferes with swallowing*

❏ *Risk of fistula formation is greatest in patients who have had both surgery and radiation therapy*
- ☐ Pack with iodoform gauze
- ☐ Allow to heal gradually over few weeks

◼ Glottic carcinoma

1. Assessment

❏ *Impairment of vocal cord motion may indicate extension of tumor into cricoarytenoid articulation and arytenoid region*

2. Treatment

❏ *Early lesions treated with equal success by radiotherapy or conservation surgery*
- ☐ When cord fixation is not needed, conservative laryngeal resection is usually treatment of choice
- ☐ Hemilaryngectomy indicated if tumor extends forward to anterior commissure or posteriorly to or beyond vocal process
- ☐ Radiotherapy is option for cure; if there is no response after reasonable dosage, therapy may be discontinued and surgery may be indicated

❑ *Advanced disease (T3 or T4) often requires total laryngectomy; any patient with obvious metastases to lateral neck nodes should undergo radical neck dissection*

  ☐ Permanent voice loss and alteration of airway occur when larynx is removed

  ▪ Establish means of communication for postoperative period prior to surgery

  ▪ Long-term options for communication include electrolarynx, esophageal speech, and voice restoration by esophageal prosthetic voice restoration

❑ *Postoperative care*

  ☐ Laryngectomy stoma care, including instructions on how to remove and clean tube and care for stoma

  ☐ Humidity is important to moisten, warm, and filter air

  ☐ Teach patients importance of mobilizing secretions by coughing, drinking adequate fluids, and instilling saline into stoma to loosen secretions, if necessary

  ☐ Hyposmia occurs in most laryngectomy patients; taste may also be affected

  ☐ Swallowing may be affected by stricture; managed by periodic dilation

  ☐ Radiation may contribute to fistula formation at suture line

  ☐ Patients should not lift heavy objects, participate in water sports, or get dust or dirt into airway when gardening or doing housework

■ Supraglottic carcinoma

1. Assessment

❑ *Generally few symptoms*

❑ *Pain may occur*

❑ *Poorly defined throat and neck discomfort during swallowing*

❑ *Referred otalgia may occur with throat pain*

❑ *Indirect laryngoscopy usually used to make diagnosis*

2. Treatment

❑ *Radiation is usually treatment of choice*

❑ *If radiation fails, total laryngectomy is usually needed as salvage procedure*

　　☐ Standard supraglottic laryngectomy consists of resection of hyoid bone, epiglottis, preepiglottic space, thyrohyoid membrane, superior half of thyroid cartilage, and false vocal cords

　　☐ Temporary tracheostomy tube is placed at surgery and removed when patient can swallow without aspirating, usually 10 to 14 days after surgery

　　☐ Patient needs to learn new method of swallowing; liquids are most difficult

■ **General treatment measures for head and neck cancers**

1. **Reconstruction: Goal is to restore function and maintain socially adequate cosmesis**
   ❏ *Myocutaneous flap*
      □ Indicated in cases where large amount of tissue has been resected and bulk is needed to reconstruct defect
      □ Flap consists of muscle, skin, and blood supply; in some cases bone or cartilage is included
      □ Pectoralis major, sternocleidomastoid, trapezius, and latissimus dorsi are muscles most often used to reconstruct head and neck defects
   ❏ *Free flap*
      □ Microvascular anastomosis used to completely remove free flap from donor site and place into recipient site
      □ Advantage of free flap is immediate functional reconstructive replacement of removed tissue
   ❏ *Deltopectoral flap*
      □ Advantage is that well-vascularized tissue from area that has not been irradiated is brought to area that has been irradiated
      □ Disadvantages include several-step procedure, and occurrence of strictures and fistulas

2. **Chemotherapy**
   ❏ *Used as*
      □ Primary chemotherapy (prior to surgery and radiation)
      □ Single-agent therapy
      □ Sequential therapy with radiation

❏ *Attempted as means of preserving structure and function of tissues*

❏ *For most head and neck cancers, chemotherapy as primary treatment has not improved survival in comparison with surgery*

3. Radiation therapy

❏ *Often used as primary therapy; also used as adjuvant therapy with surgery or chemotherapy, or both*

❏ *Treatment methods include*

  ☐ External beam radiation

  ☐ Implant therapy (*brachytherapy*)

  ▪ Use of radioactive sources placed directly into tumor

  ▪ Used to cure early-stage lesions in floor of mouth and anterior tongue

  ▪ May be used to boost tumor that has already received external beam therapy

  ▪ Radioactive seeds may be permanently implanted at surgery

  ☐ Intraoperative

  ▪ Involves delivery of single, large dose of radiation to either gross disease or tumor bed after surgical resection and during operative procedure

❏ *Hyperthermia may be combined with radiation therapy to enhance tumor response*

❏ *Increased numbers of tumor cells may be killed by combining radiation and chemotherapy*

❑ *Nursing managment*
- ☐ Mucositis
  - ▪ May appear as early as first week of treatment; usually resolves within 3 weeks after end of treatment
  - ▪ Good oral care is essential to ease discomfort and prevent infection
- ☐ *Xerostomia* (drying of oral mucosa due to loss of saliva from damage to salivary glands after radiation therapy to head and neck)
- ☐ Loss of taste (see Chap. 9 on Radiotherapy, and Chap. 21 on Integumentary Alterations for nursing care measures)

4. Management of altered airway

❑ *Tracheostomy*
- ☐ If tumor affects patient's breathing or if surgical procedure includes compromised airway, tracheostomy is necessary
- ☐ At time of surgery, cuffed tracheostomy tube is usually sutured in place
- ☐ Teach patients to suction tracheostomy tube, remove and clean inner cannula, clean tracheostoma, and apply clean dressing, as necessary
- ☐ Tracheostomy tube is removed when it is no longer needed. Slit incision is taped, and site heals over in 4 to 6 weeks

❑ *Laryngectomy*
- ☐ No longer any communication between oral cavity and lungs
- ☐ Laryngectomy stoma leads directly into lungs; mouth leads directly to stomach, with no risk of aspiration

☐ Adequate humidity is crucial; encourage adequate fluid intake to maintain fluid secretions that are easy to cough up

Suggested Readings

1. Bildstein CY: Head and neck malignancies. In Groenwald SL, Frogge MH, Goodman M, Yarbro CH (eds.): *Cancer Nursing: Principles and Practice* (3rd ed.). Boston: Jones and Bartlett, 1993, pp. 1114–1147.

2. Spiro R, Rice D: *Current Concepts in Head and Neck Cancer.* New York: American Cancer Society, 1989, p. 1.

3. Logemann J: Swallowing and communication rehabilitation. *Semin Oncol Nurs* 5:205–212, 1989.

4. Dropkin M: Coping with disfigurement and dysfunction after head and neck cancer surgery: A conceptual framework. *Semin Oncol Nurs* 5:213–219, 1989.

■ 46 ■
Hodgkin's Disease

Overview

- Hodgkin's disease (HD) accounts for 15% of malignant lymphomas and 1% of all cancers

- Incidence of HD has two peaks

1. Young adults aged 20 to 30 years

2. Adults over 45 years of age

- Etiology remains unclear

1. Infectious source has been speculated

2. Familial patterns have been noted

Approaches to Patient Care

- Assessment

1. Clinical manifestations

❏ *Enlarged lymph nodes greater than 1 cm*
  □ Painless, firm, rubbery and moveable
  □ Most located in cervical and supraclavicular areas
  □ Axillary and inguinal involvement in less than 10% of patients

❏ *Mediastinal adenopathy is common*

❏ *Constitutional symptoms, or* "B" *symptoms, are more common in advanced disease and include*
  □ Fever
  □ Malaise
  □ Night sweats
  □ Weight loss (>10% of normal body weight)
  □ Pruritus

2. Diagnostic measures

❏ *Biopsy of involved tissue*

❏ *Histologic typing and staging are necessary to determine prognosis and therapy*

❏ *HD is distinguished on histology by presence of Reed-Sternberg cell*

❏ *There are four distinct subtypes of HD*
  □ Nodular sclerosis
    ▪ More common in women than men
    ▪ Incidence between ages 15 and 34 years
    ▪ Most asymptomatic at presentation
  □ Lymphocyte-predominant
    ▪ Occurs in fourth or fifth decade of life
    ▪ Most asymptomatic at presentation
    ▪ Good prognosis

- □ Mixed cellularity
  - More common in men; wide age range
  - More than 50% of patients have B symptoms and are stage III or IV
- □ Lymphocyte-depleted
  - More common in elderly men
  - Most aggressive of four types

❑ *Staging determines extent of disease and treatment*

■ Interventions

1. **Majority of patients are curable with optimal therapy**

2. **Guidelines for treatment of HD are**

   ❑ *Radiation therapy (RT) for limited disease*

   ❑ *RT and combination chemotherapy for patients with mediastinal disease, B symptoms, and abdominal nodes*

3. **Combination therapy involves mechlorethamine, vincristine, procarbazine, and prednisone (MOPP) regimen or Adriamycin, bleomycin, vinblastine, and dacarbazine (ABVD) regimen; they may also be alternated**

   ❑ *MOPP Regimen*

Nitrogen mustard	6 mg/m^2 IV	Days 1 and 8
Vincristine (Oncovin)	1.4 mg/m^2 IV	Days 1 and 8
Procarbazine	100 mg/m^2 PO	Days 1–14
Prednisone (cycles 1 and 4 only)	40 mg/m^2 PO	Days 1–14

Repeat cycle every 28 days for minimum of six cycles. Complete remission must be documented before discontinuing therapy

❏   *ABVD Regimen*

Doxorubicin (Adriamycin)	25 mg/m² IV	Days 1 and 15
Bleomycin	10 units/m² IV	Days 1 and 15
Vinblastine	6 mg/m² IV	Days 1 and 15
Dacarbazine (DTIC)	375 mg/m² IV	Days 1 and 15

Repeat cycle every 28 days for minimum of six cycles. Complete remission must be documented before discontinuing therapy

4. **Treatment success depends on dosage and timing of therapy**

5. **If patient relapses more than 12 months after initial therapy, treat him or her with same agents**

6. **If relapse occurs less than 12 months after initial remission, patients are seldom cured; autologous bone marrow transplant may be an option**

7. **Long-term complications in cured patients**

   ❏ *Gonadal dysfunction*
     ☐ Consider reproductive counselling and sperm banking

   ❏ *Second malignancies*
     ☐ Acute nonlymphocytic leukemia most common

   ❏ *Immunologic dysfunction resulting in infections*

❑ *Herpes zoster*

❑ *Progressive radiation myelopathy*

❑ *Pneumonitis*

❑ *Pericarditis and cardiomyopathy*

8. Nurses play pivotal role in

❑ *Promoting compliance to treatment; clinical course is lengthy and toxic*

❑ *Providing emotional support*

❑ *Providing symptom management*

❑ *Rehabilitating individual to healthy lifestyle*

Suggested Readings

1. McFadden ME: Malignant lymphomas. In Groenwald SL, Frogge MH, Goodman M, Yarbro CH (eds.): *Cancer Nursing: Principles and Practice.* Boston: Jones and Bartlett, 1993, pp. 1200–1228.

2. Eyre HJ, Farver ML: Hodgkin's disease and non-Hodgkin's lymphoma. In Holleb AI, Fink DJ, Murphy GP (eds.): *Textbook of Clinical Oncology.* Atlanta: American Cancer Society, 1991, pp. 377–396.

3. Yarbro CH: Lymphomas. In Groenwald SL, Frogge MH, Goodman M, Yarbro CH (eds.): *Cancer Nursing: Principles and Practice* (2nd ed.) Boston: Jones and Bartlett, 1990, pp. 974–989.

▪ 47 ▪
Leukemia

Overview

■ Represents group of hematologic malignancies that affect bone marrow and lymph tissue

■ Occurs more frequently in adults than in children

■ Approximately one-half of cases are acute and others are chronic

■ Common types of leukemia are

1. Acute myelogenous leukemia (AML)
   ❑ *Median age at diagnosis is 50 to 60 years*

2. Acute lymphocytic leukemia (ALL)
   ❑ *More common in children*

3. Chronic myelogenous leukemia (CML)

❏ *Median age of occurrence is 49 years*
❏ *Both sexes affected*

4. Chronic lymphocytic leukemia (CLL)

❏ *Median age at diagnosis is 60 years*
❏ *More common in males*

■ **Cause is not known but common etiologic factors considered are**

1. Genetic factors

❏ *Family clustering*
❏ *Chromosomal abnormalities*

2. Radiation

3. Chemical exposure to

❏ *Benzene*
❏ *Paint*
❏ *Dye*

4. Drugs

❏ *Alkylating agents*
❏ *Chloramphenicol*
❏ *Phenylbutazone*

5. Viruses

■ **Classified according to type of cell that is predominant and location where cell maturation stopped**

1. Acute leukemia has more immature cells

2. Chronic leukemia has more mature cells that are ineffective

■ **Regulatory mechanisms that control cell numbers and growth are missing or abnormal**

■ **Manifestations are related to three factors**

1. **Increase of immature white cells in bone marrow, spleen, liver, and lymph nodes**

2. **Infiltration of these leukemic cells into body tissues**

3. **Decrease in leukocytes, thrombocytes, and erythrocytes due to crowding of bone marrow with leukemic cells**

Approaches to Patient Care

■ **Assessment of acute leukemia**

1. **Clinical manifestations**

   ❏ *Nonspecific complaints*
   - ☐ Fever
   - ☐ Weight loss
   - ☐ Fatigue

   ❏ *Recurrent infections*

   ❏ *Unexplained bleeding*
   - ☐ Bruising
   - ☐ Petechiae
   - ☐ Nosebleeds

   ❏ *Progressive anemia with shortness of breath, splenomegaly, weakness, and fatigue*

   ❏ *Joint pain*

❏ *Neurologic complaints*
  ☐ Headache
  ☐ Vomiting
  ☐ Visual disturbances

2. Diagnostic measures

❏ *Must differentiate between AML and ALL since treatment and prognosis are very different*

❏ *Bone marrow biopsy and aspirate for definitive diagnosis*

❏ *Ninety percent of patients have blast cells in peripheral blood smear*

❏ *Serum chemistries may reveal hyperuricemia*

❏ *Chromosome analysis to determine classification*

■ Interventions

1. Treatment of AML

❏ *Goal is to eradicate leukemic stem cell*

❏ *Complete remission (CR) is restoration of normal blood counts and less than 5% blast cells*

❏ *Course of therapy is divided into two stages*
  ☐ Induction therapy
    ▪ Cytosine arabinoside continuously for 7 days
    ▪ Anthracycline (e.g., daunorubicin, doxorubicin) for 3 days

- Bone marrow biopsy on day 14; if leukemic cells are present, begin a second course

- Twenty percent of AML patients remain in CR; the rest relapse in 1 to 2 years

☐ Postremission therapy

- *Consolidation:* Give high doses of induction therapy drugs for 1 to 2 courses

- *Intensification:* Give different drugs after CR

❏ *Patients who relapse after induction or postremission therapy have 30% to 60% chance of second remission*

❏ *Bone marrow transplant (BMT) for AML is controversial*

2. Treatment of ALL

❏ *Goal is to eradicate leukemic cells from marrow and lymph tissue and residual disease from central nervous system (CNS)*

❏ *Treatment involves drugs that are more selective to lymphoblasts and less toxic to normal cells*

❏ *Long-term survival more favorable with ALL than AML*

❏ *Course of therapy is divided into three stages*

☐ Induction therapy

- Vincristine, prednisone, and L-asparaginase plus an anthracycline

- Only 70% to 75% of adults achieve CR

☐ CNS prophylaxis

- Intracranial radiation and intrathecal methotrexate

□ Postremission therapy

- Same drugs as with induction;
  methotrexate and 6-mercaptopurine may
  be added

- Maintenance therapy continues for 2 to 3
  years

❏ *Outlook is poor for patients who relapse
during therapy*

❏ *There is better prognosis with BMT if it is
performed during first remission*

■ Assessment of CML

1. Clinical manifestations

❏ *Twenty percent of CML patients have no
symptoms at diagnosis*

❏ *Left upper quadrant pain, abdominal fullness,
early satiety are related to massive
splenomegaly*

❏ *Malaise, fatigue*

❏ *Fever*

❏ *Weight loss*

❏ *Bone and joint pain*

2. Diagnostic studies may reveal

❏ *White blood cell (WBC) count
> 100,000/mm^3*

❏ *Anemia*

❏ *Thrombocytosis*

❏ *Philadelphia (Ph^1) chromosome*

■ Interventions

1. Treatment of CML

❑ *Only chance for cure is ablation of Ph^1 chromosome by high-dose chemotherapy and BMT; only 25% of patients have this option*

❑ *Natural course of CML has two phases*
   □ Chronic phase
      ▪ Treatment with oral busulfan or hydroxyurea
      ▪ Treatment does not prevent progression to terminal phase
   □ Terminal phase

❑ *Blastic transformation can be detected 3 to 4 months before clinical signs are evident*

❑ *Blast crisis requires intensive chemotherapy, similar to agents used for AML*

❑ *Median survival after onset of terminal phase is 3 months*

■ Assessment of CLL

1. Clinical manifestations

❑ *Recurrent infections (skin and respiratory)*
❑ *Splenomegaly*
❑ *Lymphadenopathy in advanced disease*

2. Diagnostic studies may reveal

❑ *WBC > 20,000/mm^3 in early disease*

❑ *WBC > 100,000/mm^3 in advanced disease*

❏ *Hypogammaglobulinemia*

❏ *Bone marrow biopsy needed for definitive diagnosis*

Interventions

1. Treatment of CLL

❏ *Observe asymptomatic patients*

❏ *Treat symptomatic patients with oral chlorambucil or cyclophosphamide*

❏ *Give corticosteroids to control leukocytosis*

❏ *Perform splenectomy and radiation therapy when patients no longer respond to chemotherapy and corticosteroids*

❏ *Give combination therapy (cyclophosphamide, vincristine, doxorubicin, prednisone) for advanced disease*

❏ *Give fludarabine to patients who are refractory to alkylating agents*

Supportive care interventions

1. Supportive therapies may improve quality of survival

2. Nurse plays key role in patient and family education, physical care, psychosocial support, and symptom management

3. Symptom management of common side effects

❏ *Neutropenia*

☐ Absolute neutrophil count less than 1000/mm^3 is common

☐ Sixty percent of leukemia patients develop infection

☐ Common sites of infection are
   - Pharynx, esophagus
   - Anorectal area
   - Sinuses
   - Lungs
   - Skin

☐ Usual signs and symptoms of infection may be absent due to lack of inflammatory response

☐ Fever more than 100° F requires cultures of blood, urine, sputum, and intravenous sites

☐ Empiric antibiotic therapy is used until organism is identified

☐ Give amphotericin B for life-threatening fungal infections and if fever continues 5 to 7 days after start of antibiotic therapy

☐ Give prophylactic fluconazole to prevent disseminated infections

☐ To prevent infection
   - Maintain patient's skin integrity, sleep, and nutrition
   - Decrease invasive procedures
   - Provide private room, restrict visitors
   - Patient should avoid uncooked foods
   - Patient and caregivers should practice meticulous hand washing
   - Do not allow plants or fresh flowers

  ☐ Adminster colony-stimulating factors to shorten period of neutropenia

❏ *Erythrocytopenia*

  ☐ Give transfusions of red blood cells if there is sudden blood loss or symptomatic anemia

❏ *Thrombocytopenia*

  ☐ There is potential bleeding if platelets are < 50,000/mm^3

  ☐ There is spontaneous bleeding if platelets are < 20,000/mm^3

  ☐ First signs of bleeding may be

   ▪ Petechiae or ecchymoses on mucous membranes or skin of dependent limbs

   ▪ Oozing from gums, nose or intravenous site

  ☐ Give random donor platelets to keep platelet count > 20,000/mm^3

  ☐ Measures to prevent bleeding

   ▪ Maintain patient's skin integrity

   ▪ Prevent trauma

   ▪ Patient should avoid medications with anticoagulant effects

   ▪ Patient should take stool softeners to prevent straining

4. **Nursing care plan should anticipate complications of disease or therapy**

❏ *Leukostasis*

  ☐ Patients at risk have WBC > 50,000/mm^3

  ☐ Occurs more often in ALL

- □ Intracerebral hemorrhage most common manifestation

- □ Reduce burden of cells by
  - High-dose chemotherapy
  - Leukapheresis
  - Cranial radiation

❏ *Disseminated intravascular coagulation (DIC)*

- □ May occur with any acute leukemia

- □ Correction of DIC depends on successful treatment of leukemia

- □ Nursing care focuses on
  - Prevention of injury
  - Administration of prescribed therapy
  - Monitoring of lab results

❏ *Oral complications*

- □ Result of disease or therapy
- □ Gingival hypertrophy
- □ Stomatitis
- □ Provide routine oral care

❏ *Cerebellar toxicity*

- □ Associated with high-dose cytosine arabinoside (HDCA) (>3 g/m^2)

- □ Increased risk in patients older than 50 years

- □ Ataxia and nystagmus are early signs

- □ Difficulty with speech and rapid movements are late signs

- □ Toxicity is irreversible if not detected early

- □ Complete neurologic assessment before each HDCA

Suggested Readings

1. Wujcik D: Leukemia. In Groenwald SL, Frogge MH, Goodman M, Yarbro CH (eds.): *Cancer Nursing: Principles and Practice* (3rd ed.). Boston: Jones and Bartlett, 1993, pp. 1149–1173.

2. Oniboni AC: Infection in the neutropenic patient. *Semin Oncol Nurs* 6:50–60, 1990.

3. Levinson JA, Lesko LM: Psychiatric aspects of adult leukemia. *Semin Oncol Nurs* 6:76–83, 1990.

4. McNally JL, Somerville ET, Miaskowski C, Rostad M (eds.): *Guidelines for Cancer Nursing Practice* (2nd ed.) Philadelphia: WB Saunders, 1991.

▪ 48 ▪
Liver Cancer

Overview

- ■ Leading cause of death in Africa and Asia

- ■ In U.S., limited number of cases develop

- ■ Five times more prevalent among men than women

- ■ Average age of onset is 60 to 70 years

- ■ Unusual clinical and pathologic features

- ■ Disseminates early

- ■ No specific treatment effectively controls disease

- ■ Risk factors

1. Cirrhosis
   - ❏ *Alcohol-induced*

❏ *Resulting from poor nutrition*
❏ *Posthepatic*
❏ *Hemochromatosis*

2. **Hepatitis B or C**

3. **Malnutrition**

4. **Aflatoxin**

5. **Mycotoxin**

6. **Thorotrast biliary contrast medium**

■ **Tumors may be primary or secondary tumors metastasized from other sites**

■ **Differentiating whether tumor is primary or secondary is critical treatment issue**

1. **Primary liver cancers are of two types**

   ❏ *Ninety percent are hepatocellular*

   ❏ *Seven percent are cholangiocarcinoma*

   ❏ *Typically originate in right lobe*

   ❏ *May be multicentric in origin or start with single focus*

   ❏ *Usually soft, highly vascular, and diffluent with stroma*

   ❏ *Often well differentiated with clearly defined margins*

2. **Secondary liver cancers**

   ❏ *Twenty times more likely to occur than primary tumor*

❏ *Liver is repository for metastatic deposits from nearly all sites*

❏ *Metastases may occur as single mass or as multiple masses*

❏ *Metastases are frequently from*
  ◻ Lung   ◻ Kidney
  ◻ Breast   ◻ Intestinal tract

■ **Progression of disease occurs by direct extension within and around liver**

■ **Tumors typically alter liver bloodflow, receive their blood supply from hepatic artery, and drain via hepatic vein**

■ **Occlusion of vessels is common**

■ **In advanced disease**

1. **Liver failure and hemorrhage are complications leading to death**

2. **Tamponade within liver can lead to necrosis and rupture or hemorrhage**

3. **Prognosis is poor, with overall 5-year survival of 5%**

4. **If untreated, death occurs in 6 to 8 weeks**

Approaches to Care

■ **Assessment**

1. **Clinical manifestations**

   ❏ *Can grow to huge proportions before detected*

❏ *Common signs are*
  □ Right upper quadrant pain that is dull and aching
  □ Continuous pain that interrupts sleep and is aggravated by activity or lying on right side
  □ Profound, progressive weakness and fatigue
  □ Fullness in epigastrium
  □ Constipation or diarrhea
  □ Anorexia or weight loss
  □ Ascites and signs of portal hypertension
  □ Hematemesis

2. Diagnostic measures

❏ *Definitive diagnostic tool is tissue diagnosis*

❏ *Physical examination may reveal painful, enlarged liver*

❏ *Other diagnostic studies*
  □ Abdominal x-ray to show displacement or deformity of organs
  □ Ultrasound of abdomen
  □ CT of abdomen and lungs
  □ MRI is as effective as CT
  □ Radionuclide scanning outlines tumors in liver
  □ Selective hepatic arteriography shows vascular abnormalities in liver blood supply
  □ Hematologic profiles
  □ Liver function tests
  □ Tumor marker alpha-fetoprotein (AFP)
  □ Needle biopsy (only if tumor is unresectable)

■ Interventions

1. Choice of treatment depends on

- ❏ *Whether tumor is primary or secondary*
- ❏ *Type and extent of tumor*
- ❏ *Concomitant diseases*
- ❏ *Liver function*
- ❏ *Patient status*

2. Pretreatment therapy

- ❏ *Anemia, clotting deficits, fluid and electrolyte abnormalities should be corrected*

- ❏ *Vitamin A, C, D, and B complex can reduce effect of jaundice*

- ❏ *Pruritus can be relieved with good hygiene and by avoiding products that dry skin and using oil-based lotions, antihistamines, and cholestyramine*

- ❏ *Nutritional improvement is critical*

3. Treatment

- ❏ *Cure is objective for*
  - ☐ Primary liver cancer that is localized
  - ☐ Solitary mass without evidence of regional lymph node involvement
  - ☐ Secondary tumors that are solitary or well defined

- ❏ *Control is objective if tumor is*
  - ☐ Multicentric
  - ☐ Metastatic
  - ☐ Secondary

❏ *Surgery*

   ☐ Surgical risk is directly related to degree of cirrhosis

   ☐ If noncancerous lobe is normal or mildly cirrhotic, lobectomy can be undertaken

   ☐ If cirrhosis is advanced, left lobectomy can be undertaken; right lobectomy can be life-threatening

   ☐ Local resection, ultrasound-guided cryosurgery, or laser surgery may be possible

   ☐ Hepatic artery occlusion or embolization can deprive tumor of its blood supply and necrose it

   ☐ Postoperative care is concerned with

      ■ Hemorrhage
      ■ Infection
      ■ Subphrenic abscess
      ■ Atelectasis
      ■ Clotting defects
      ■ Biliary fistula
      ■ Transient metabolic changes
      ■ Pneumonia
      ■ Portal hypertension

❏ *Chemotherapy*

   ☐ May be treatment of choice if surgery is not option

   ☐ Regional therapy

      ■ Isolated to liver
      ■ Provides high concentration of drug directly to tumor
      ■ Dose limitations are toxicity-related

       Drugs include

         5-Fluorouracil

Cisplatin

Doxorubicin

Mitomycin-C

Nitrogen mustard

Methotrexate

- ☐ Intraperitoneal chemotherapy
    - ▪ Used successfully
    - ▪ Trials are limited in number

- ❏ *Radiation therapy*
    - ☐ Limited to palliation
    - ☐ Doses range from 1900 to 3100 cGy over 2 to 20 days
    - ☐ Major side effects are nausea, vomiting, anorexia, fatigue

- ❏ *Supportive therapy*
    - ☐ Most individuals die within 6 months of diagnosis
    - ☐ Advanced disease manifests
        - ▪ Hepatic failure
        - ▪ Infection
        - ▪ Pain
        - ▪ Weakness
        - ▪ Severe ascites
        - ▪ Bleeding
        - ▪ Weight loss
        - ▪ Pneumonia
    - ☐ Pain is most difficult to manage
        - ▪ Worsens at night and is severe
        - ▪ Aggravated by movement
        - ▪ See Chapter 27 for specific interventions

Suggested Readings

1. Frogge MH. Gastrointestinal cancer: Esophagus, stomach, liver, and pancreas. In Groenwald SL, Frogge MH, Goodman M, Yarbro CH (eds.): *Cancer Nursing: Principles and Practice* (3rd ed.). Boston: Jones and Bartlett, 1993, pp. 1022–1029.

2. Ahlgren JD, Wanebo HJ, Hill MC: Hepatocellular carcinoma. In Ahlgren JD, Macdonald JS (eds.): *Gastrointestinal Oncology.* Philadelphia: Lippincott, 1992, pp. 417–436.

3. Cady B, Stone MD, McDermott WV, et al: Technical and biological factors in disease-free survival after hepatic resection for colorectal cancer metastases. *Arch Surg* 127:561–569, 1992.

4. Patt YZ, Mavligit GM: Arterial chemotherapy in the management of colorectal cancer: An overview. *Semin Oncol* 18(5):478–490, 1991.

Lung Cancer

Overview

1. Most common cancer killer

2. Eighty-five percent of cases are preventable if cigarette smoking is eliminated

3. Five-year survival is poor

4. Occurs after repeated exposures to substances that cause irritation and inflammation

5. Major risk factors are
   - ❏ *Tobacco smoke*
   - ❏ *Passive smoking*
   - ❏ *Air pollution*
   - ❏ *Occupational exposure to toxic substances*
   - ❏ *Radon*
   - ❏ *Low vitamin A levels*

6. Two major histologic classes of lung cancer are

❏ *Non–small-cell lung cancer (NSCLC)*
  ☐ Squamous cell carcinoma
    ▪ Associated with cigarette smoking
    ▪ Accounts for 30% of all lung cancers
    ▪ Slow growing and longer survival
  ☐ Adenocarcinomas
    ▪ Most common of lung cancers
    ▪ Most frequent type found in women
    ▪ Metastasis is common, especially to the brain
  ☐ Large-cell carcinomas
    ▪ Accounts for 10% to 15% of lung cancers

❏ *Small-cell lung cancer (SCLC)*
  ☐ Associated with smoking
  ☐ Comprises 30% of all lung cancers
  ☐ High growth rate and metastasize early

Approaches to Patient Care

▣ Assessment

1. Clinical manifestations
  ❏ *Cough*
  ❏ *Chest pain*
  ❏ *Dyspnea*
  ❏ *Wheezing*
  ❏ *Hemoptysis*
  ❏ *Anorexia*
  ❏ *Weight loss*
  ❏ *Fatigue*
  ❏ *Hoarseness*
  ❏ *Dysphagia*

❏ *Chest or shoulder pain*
❏ *Paraneoplastic syndromes*

2. Diagnostic measures

❏ *Rarely diagnosed in early stage*
❏ *Sputum cytology*
❏ *Chest x-ray*
❏ *Bronchoscopy*
❏ *Percutaneous needle biopsy*
❏ *Mediastinoscopy*
❏ *CT and MRI*

▓ Interventions

1. NSCLC

❏ *Extent of disease determines treatment and prognosis*

❏ *Surgery*

☐ Complete surgical resection is only chance for cure

☐ Only 20% to 25% of NSCLC patients qualify for complete surgical resection

☐ Lobectomy or pneumonectomy are surgical procedures for localized disease

❏ *Radiation therapy (RT)*

☐ For patients who are not surgical candidates; however, most NSCLCs have poor radiosensitivity

☐ Contraindicated in patients in poor general condition

❏ *Chemotherapy*
  ☐ NSCLCs less sensitive to chemotherapy
  ☐ Cisplatin and RT for inoperable patients has increased survival 4 to 6 months

2. SCLC

❏ *Prognostic indicators are extent of disease, performance status, weight loss, and response to therapy*

❏ *Combination chemotherapy with or without RT is standard treatment*

❏ *Chemotherapy combinations have included*
  ☐ Cyclophosphamide   ☐ Etoposide
  ☐ Doxorubicin   ☐ Cisplatin
  ☐ Vincristine   ☐ Ifosfamide

❏ *High doses produce better response*

❏ *RT to chest with chemotherapy has reduced intrathoracic relapse*

❏ *Prophylactic brain irradiation has been used*

3. Symptom management

❏ *Distressing physical symptoms include*
  ☐ Cough   ☐ Hemoptysis
  ☐ Pain   ☐ Wheezing
  ☐ Dyspnea

❏ *Pulmonary fibrosis may occur as result of RT and chemotherapy*

❏ *Psychosocial issues and dilemmas include*
  ☐ Quality of life
  ☐ Social isolation as result of symptoms
  ☐ Limited survival
  ☐ Family disruptions

4. Because of poor survival, nurses coordinate and provide palliative interventions

Suggested Readings

1. Elpern EH: Lung cancer. In Groenwald SL, Frogge MH, Goodman M, Yarbro CH (eds.): *Cancer Nursing: Principles and Practice* (3rd ed.). Boston: Jones and Bartlett, 1993, pp. 1174–1199.

2. Risser NL: The key to prevention of lung cancer. *Semin Oncol Nurs* 3:228–236, 1987.

3. Foote M, Sexton DL, Pawlik L: Dyspnea: A distressing symptom in lung cancer. *Oncol Nurs Forum* 13:25–31, 1986.

4. Bernhard J, Ganz PA: Psychosocial issues in lung cancer patients. *Chest* 99:480–485, 1991.

■ 50 ■
Multiple Myeloma

Overview

■ Most common of plasma cell disorders

■ Characterized by overproduction of specific immunoglobulin, designated IgM or M protein

■ About 80% to 90% of multiple myeloma patients have aberrant M protein in serum

■ Although excessive amount of immunoglobulin is produced, M protein is unable to produce antibody necessary for maintaining humoral immunity

■ Affects hematologic, skeletal, renal, and nervous systems

■ Represents 1% of hematologic malignancies

■ **Onset is late**

■ **Peak incidence is between 50 and 70 years of age**

■ **More common among blacks than whites (14:1)**

■ **Male dominance in all groups**

■ **Once symptoms present, median survival is 7 months; survival can extend to 2 to 3 years with standard therapy**

■ **Risk factors**

1. **Genetic linkage**

2. **Chronic low-level exposure to radiation**

3. **Chronic antigenic stimulation (infection, allergy)**

Approaches to Care

■ **Assessment**

1. **Clinical manifestations**

   ❏ *Multiple myeloma has a long prodromal, indolent, or asymptomatic period. Once symptoms appear, systemic therapy begins*

   ❏ *Skeletal involvement*
   □ Sixty-eight percent to 80% of patients present with destructive, painful osteolytic lesions

- ☐ Hypercalcemia
- ☐ Pathologic fractures with acute and chronic pain
- ☐ Decreased mobility
- ☐ Diminished ability in activities of daily living
- ☐ Bony lesions can be of three types
    - ▪ Solitary osteolytic lesion
    - ▪ Diffuse osteoporosis
    - ▪ Multiple discrete osteolytic lesions ("punched out" or "cannon ball" lesions)
- ☐ Eventually skeletal involvement can lead to
    - ▪ Compression fractures of spine
    - ▪ Refractory hypercalcemia
    - ▪ Death from neurologic sequelae or severe hypercalcemia

❏ *Infection*
- ☐ Fifty percent to 70% of patients die from bacterial infections
- ☐ Most common sites are respiratory and urinary tract
- ☐ Biphasic pattern is common
    - ▪ *Streptococcus pneumoniae* and *Haemophilus influenzae* occur early in disease
    - ▪ Nonencapsulated gram-negative bacilli occur later
    - ▪ Mechanisms of infection
        Deficiency in immunoglobulin
        Neutropenia associated with bone marrow suppression
        Qualitative defects in neutrophil and complement function

❏ *Bone marrow involvement*

☐ Normocytic, normochromic anemia occurs in more than 60% of patients at initial diagnosis

☐ Red blood cell destruction caused by M protein coating erythrocytes

☐ Bleeding caused by M protein's effect on clotting factors or by coating of platelets with immunoglobulins

❏ *Renal insufficiency*

☐ Fifty percent of patients develop insufficiency

☐ Fifteen percent die from renal failure

☐ Intrinsic lesion associated with renal failure is called *myeloma kidney*

☐ Bence Jones proteins develop

☐ Amyloid deposits can cause lesions

❏ *Other manifestations*

☐ Hypercalcemia

☐ Hyperuricemia occurs with large tumor burdens

☐ Dehydration

❏ *Hyperviscosity syndrome*

☐ Caused by high concentration of proteins that increases serum viscosity and results in vascular sludging

☐ Clinical signs

- Blurred vision
- Irritability
- Headache
- Drowsiness
- Confusion

2. Diagnostic measures

❏ *Bone marrow biopsy to check percentage of plasma cells*

- ❏ *Serum protein electrophoresis to check for presence of M protein*
- ❏ *Serum chemistry for hypercalcemia or renal function*
- ❏ *Complete blood count for anemia, thrombocytopenia*
- ❏ *Skeletal survey for bone lesions*
- ❏ *Staging of multiple myeloma integrates clinical and laboratory findings*
- ❏ *Durie-Salmon system of stages I to III is commonly used*

▪ Interventions

1. **Patients with indolent, asymptomatic multiple myeloma are usually not treated**

2. **Once symptoms occur, standard therapy is initiated**

3. **Chemotherapy is used with onset of symptoms**
   - ❏ *Melphalan and prednisone are standard*
     - ☐ Response rate is 24 to 36 months
     - ☐ Melphalan 0.25 mg/kg/day for 4 days along with prednisone 2 mg/kg/day for 4 days is given every 4 weeks
     - ☐ Monitor patient closely for signs of renal impairment
     - ☐ Bone marrow suppressive effects can be cumulative in older adults

❏ *Other common protocol is vincristine, doxorubicin, and dexamethasone (VAD)*
  ☐ Vincristine 0.4 mg/24-hour infusion for 4 days; doxorubicin 9 mg/m^2/continuous infusion for 4 days; and dexamethasone 40 mg are given on alternating schedules
  ☐ Clinicians must monitor
    ▪ Total dose of doxorubicin
    ▪ Signs of steroid toxicity
      Severe dyspepsia
      Fluid and sodium retention
      Myopathy
      Pancreatitis
      Hyperglycemia
      Psychosis
    ▪ Signs of neurologic toxicity
    ▪ Bone marrow suppression
    ▪ Hepatic toxicity

❏ *If drug resistance emerges, cyclophosphamide can be used*

❏ *Thirty percent to 40% of patients will respond to first-line therapy; second-line therapies are commonly used as result*

4. Interferon
❏ *Stimulates host cells to affect tumor cells*

❏ *Has been used following standard therapy of 12 courses of induction chemotherapy to prolong response and survival*

5. Radiation
❏ *Used to palliate bone lesions and control pain*

❑ *Multiple myeloma is highly radioresponsive*

❑ *Fractionated doses are given (2000–2400 cGy) over 2 to 3 weeks*

❑ *Hemibody irradiation has been used for refractory myeloma*

6. **Bone marrow transplantation has been attempted. Technical difficulties in purging myeloma from marrow limits its use**

7. **Treatment-related leukemia**

❑ *Sequela of treating myeloma*

❑ *Cause is considered to be prolonged exposure to alkylating agents*

❑ *Occurs in 20% of patients*

❑ *Myelodysplastic syndrome is first sign*

❑ *Can be treated with standard therapy for acute nonlymphocytic leukemia*

8. **Nursing management**

❑ *Pain is usually due to bony involvement. In addition to standard approaches, positioning, braces, supports, and massages can help*

❑ *Mental status changes can result from hypercalcemia, hyperviscosity, or drug toxicity; closely assess patient to prevent injury*

❑ *Infection is leading cause of death. Early recognition and prevention of infection and bleeding are needed*

❑ *Provide respiratory care measures to prevent pooling of secretions and increase gas exchange*

❑ *Due to decreased physical activity and medications, constipation is common; assess patient's activity changes and dietary intake*

❑ *Prevent or quickly reverse renal insufficiency by providing adequate hydration, administration of allopurinol, and close monitoring for signs of urinary tract infection*

Suggested Readings

1. Sheridan CA: Multiple myeloma. In Groenwald SL, Frogge MH, Goodman M, Yarbro CH (eds.): *Cancer Nursing: Principles and Practice* (3rd ed.). Boston: Jones and Bartlett, 1993, pp. 1229–1237.

2. Wiernik PH (ed.): *Neoplastic Diseases of the Blood.* New York: Churchill-Livingstone, 1991.

3. Duffy TP: The many pitfalls of diagnosis of myeloma. *N Engl J Med* 326(6):394–396, 1992.

4. Bubley GJ, Schnipper LE: Multiple myeloma. In Holleb AI (ed.): *American Cancer Society Textbook of Clinical Oncology.* Atlanta: ACS, 1991, pp. 397–409.

▪ 51 ▪
Non-Hodgkin's Lymphoma

Overview

- Incidence of non-Hodgkin's lymphoma (NHL) is escalating and is now fifth most common cancer in U.S.

- Nearly six times more frequent than HD and death rate is 13 times greater

- Incidence is higher in males and white population

- Average age of occurrence is fifth decade

- Variety of etiologic factors have been implicated

1. Viral infections
2. Genetic abnormalities
3. Exposure to pesticides, fertilizers, chemicals

Approaches to Patient Care

■ Assessment

1. Clinical manifestations

❏ *Can involve almost any organ or tissue*

❏ *Eighty percent of patients present with advanced disease (stage III or IV) reflected by*

☐ Painless, generalized lymphadenopathy

☐ "B" symptoms
   - Fever
   - Night sweats
   - Weight loss

☐ Gastrointestinal symptoms
   - Pain
   - Abdominal mass
   - Anorexia

☐ Lung infiltration
   - Cough
   - Dyspnea
   - Chest pain
   - Pleural effusion

☐ Superior vena cava syndrome

☐ Bone, liver, brain manifestations

2. Diagnostic measures

❏ *Biopsy confirms histopathology*

❏ *Staging work-up determines extent of disease, tumor mass, and potential complications*

❏ *NHL occurs in many locations and requires numerous studies for staging*

■ Interventions

1. Treatment depends on histology, extent of disease, and performance status

❑ *Low-grade lymphomas*
   □ Occur in older individuals
   □ Occur equally in males and females
   □ Majority of patients are asymptomatic
   □ Usual presenting problem is painless lymphadenopathy
   □ Slow growing with median survival of 7 to 9 years
   □ Treatment includes irradiation, single-agent chemotherapy, or combination chemotherapy

❑ *Intermediate-grade lymphomas*
   □ *Follicular* NHL
      ■ Aggressive clinical course
      ■ Most patients have advanced disease
   □ *Diffuse* patterns of NHL
      ■ Disease limited to one side of diaphragm
      ■ Occur mostly in adults
      ■ Nodal and extranodal involvement
      ■ If untreated, survival less than 2 years
   □ Treatment includes combination chemotherapy and irradiation

❑ *High-grade lymphomas*
   □ *Immunoblastic*
      ■ Occurs in adults older than 50 years
      ■ Anemia and B symptoms are common
      ■ High incidence of cutaneous disease
      ■ Poor response to chemotherapy and poor survival rate

- ☐ Lymphoblastic
  - ■ Occurs in adolescents and young adults
  - ■ More predominant in men than in women
  - ■ Majority of patients present with mediastinal mass
  - ■ Lymph node involvement and bone lesions
  - ■ Rapid, progressive disease
- ☐ *Non-Burkitt's* lymphoma
  - ■ Uncommon; median age is 34 years
  - ■ Lymph node and extranodal presentation
  - ■ Treatment is generally ineffective and survival is approximately 1 year
- ☐ Aggressive combination chemotherapy is treatment for high-grade lymphomas
- ☐ Autologous bone marrow transplant may be option for nonresponsive high-grade lymphomas

2. **Nursing care related to radiation and chemotherapeutic side effects is covered in chapters 9 and 10**

3. **Delayed toxicities vary from minor to severe problems**

4. **Nurses play pivotal role in**
   - ❏ *Providing emotional support*
   - ❏ *Providing symptom management*
   - ❏ *Rehabilitating cured patient to return to healthy lifestyle*

Suggested Readings

1. McFadden ME: Malignant lymphomas. In Groenwald SL, Frogge MH, Goodman M, Yarbro CH (eds.): *Cancer Nursing: Principles and Practice* (3rd ed.). Boston: Jones and Bartlett, 1993, pp. 1200–1228.

2. Rahr VA, Tucker R: Non-Hodgkin's lymphoma: Understanding the disease. *Cancer Nurs* 13:56–91, 1990.

3. Yarbro CH: Lymphomas. In Groenwald SL, Frogge MH, Goodman M, Yarbro CH (eds.): *Cancer Nursing: Principles and Practice* (2nd ed.). Boston: Jones and Bartlett, 1990, pp. 974–989.

■ 52 ■
Ovarian Cancer

Overview

■ Most common cause of death from gynecologic cancers

■ Fifth leading cause of death overall in women in U.S.

■ Poor survival rate of 30% to 35% has been unchanged for 30 years due to

1. Late diagnosis

2. Lack of curative treatments

3. Inability to identify a high-risk group

4. Unknown etiology

■ In 1993, there were about 22,000 new cases and 13,000 deaths from ovarian cancer

■ An estimated 1 of every 71 women will develop the disease

■ **Occurs mostly between 55 and 59 years of age**

■ **Risk factors**

1. **Environmental factors**
   ❏ *High educational level*
   ❏ *High socioeconomic level*
   ❏ *Delayed childbearing pattern*

2. **Hormonal, menstrual, reproductive factors**
   ❏ *Nulliparity*

   ❏ *First pregnancy after 35 years of age*

   ❏ *Incessant ovulation (uninterrupted by pregnancy, lactation, contraceptives)*

   ❏ *Early menarche*

   ❏ *Late menopause*

   ❏ *Hormonal therapy*

3. **Dietary factors**
   ❏ *High-fat diet*

4. **Hereditary factors**
   ❏ *Family history of ovarian cancer*
   ❏ *Family history of breast cancer*

■ **Epithelial tumors constitute 80% to 90% of ovarian cancers**

1. **Tumors of low malignant potential, which represent 15% of epithelial tumors, are distinct entities characterized by**
   ❏ *Cellular proliferation*
   ❏ *No invasive properties*
   ❏ *Favorable prognosis*

2. **Histologic grade is important predictor of response and survival, especially stages I to II**

■ **Seventy-five percent of ovarian cancer patients have metastatic disease at diagnosis**

■ **Metastatic routes include**

1. **Invading stromal tissue**

2. **Penetrating capsule of ovary**

3. **Commonly spreading by direct extension to adjacent organs: Uterus, bladder, rectosigmoid, perineum**

4. **Peritoneal seeding: Cells exfoliate and are carried to surfaces of organs within peritoneum**

5. **Lymphatic spread**

■ **Death is often secondary to intraabdominal tumor dissemination that produces bowel and mesentery malfunction and alteration**

Approaches to Care

■ **Assessment**

1. **Clinical manifestations**
   ❑ *No typical early manifestations*
   ❑ *Abdominal fullness*
   ❑ *Discomfort*
   ❑ *Vague symptoms*

2. Diagnostic measures

❑ *Routine pelvic examination*

❑ *Transvaginal ultrasound*

❑ *Transvaginal color flow imaging (experimental)*

❑ *Barium enema*

❑ *Proctosigmoidoscopy and gastrointestinal series*

❑ *Chest x-ray*

❑ *Ultrasound*

❑ *CT scan*

❑ *MRI for small lesions*

❑ *Surgical staging and debulking*

Interventions

1. Initial therapy involves surgical staging and cytoreduction

❑ *Surgical staging involves*
  ☐ Evaluation of all peritoneal surfaces
  ☐ Evaluation of subdiaphragmatic surfaces
  ☐ Multiple biopsies
  ☐ Palpation of all abdominal organs and surfaces

❑ *Cytoreduction involves removing visible tumor to extent possible*

❑ *Stage I disease (15%–20% of patients)*
  ☐ Has 90% survival rate

- □ Beyond surgery, usually no additional therapy is given

- □ Adjuvant pelvic irradiation or chemotherapy offers no distinct advantage

❏ *Stage II disease (tumor extends to peritoneal organs) is treated following cytoreduction with*
  - □ Intraperitoneal chromic phosphate (^{32}P)
  - □ Whole-abdominal radiation
  - □ Single-agent chemotherapy
  - □ Platinum-based combination chemotherapy

❏ *Stage III and IV disease*
  - □ Requires more aggressive cytoreductive surgery and adjuvant therapy

  - □ Platinum-based combination chemotherapy

  - □ Whole-abdominal and pelvic radiation

  - □ Survival rates are comparable for chemotherapy and radiation; morbidity is greater with radiation

2. **Recurrent or persistent disease treatment approaches are of limited benefit and duration of response. Treatments include**

   ❏ *Second-look surgery is performed on those with complete clinical response following full-course chemotherapy*
     - □ To determine if therapy should stop
     - □ To assess response and change therapy
     - □ To perform secondary cytoreductive surgery

   ❏ *Tumor-associated antigens are not specific for ovarian cancer*
     - □ Carbohydrate antigen (CA)-125 is used to supplement standard methods of disease monitoring

□ CA-19–9 is used in combination with CA-125 to correlate response

❑ *Chemotherapy is mainstay for adjuvant treatment*

□ Single agents

▪ Cisplatin is most effective single agent

▪ Responses are also effected with ifosfamide, diaziquone, etoposide, and mitomycin

□ Combination chemotherapy has extensive use. Protocols of two to four agents typically include

▪ Hexamethylmelamine
▪ Cyclophosphamide
▪ Methotrexate
▪ 5-Fluorouracil
▪ Cisplatin
▪ Doxorubicin
▪ Carboplatin
▪ Taxol

□ Cisplatin, carboplatin, and taxol have generated much interest among researchers to determine effective recurrent disease protocol

□ Taxol has produced 30% response rate in previously treated patients

□ Drug resistance can result in death from chemotherapy-refractory disease

▪ Debulking surgeries to reduce tumor burden to less than 1 cm also reduce potential for development of multidrug resistance

□ Intraperitoneal chemotherapy

▪ Benefits patients who have minimal disease after systemic therapy or high-grade tumors, or both

▪ Is delivered via semipermanent dialysis catheter or implanted port system into abdominal cavity

- Large volumes of chemotherapy can be administered
  □ Hormone therapy
    - Tamoxifen has been investigated as second-line therapy for chemotherapy-refractory disease

❏ *Radiotherapy*
  □ ^{32}P can be administered by intraperitoneal infusion to produce even distribution of agent throughout abdomen
  □ External beam therapy is limited by bulk of tumor to be treated
  □ If tumor is less than 2 cm, equivalent results are achieved with radiation or chemotherapy

❏ *Biologic therapy*
  □ Includes monoclonal antibodies, adoptive cellular immunotherapy, and interferon
  □ Agents remain in abdominal cavity for prolonged periods
  □ Agents have manageable toxicities

❏ *Management of side effects is reviewed in Chapters 10 and 11*

Suggested Readings

1. Walczak J, Klemm PR: Gynecologic cancers. In Groenwald SL, Frogge MH, Goodman M, Yarbro CH (eds.): *Cancer Nursing: Principles and Practice* (3rd ed.). Boston: Jones and Bartlett, 1993, pp. 1065–1113.

2. Piver MS, Baker TR, Piedmonte M, Sandecki AM: Epidemiology and etiology of ovarian cancer. *Semin Oncol* 18(3):177–185, 1991.

3. Eriksson JH, Walczak JR: Ovarian cancer. *Semin Oncol Nurs* 6:214–227, 1990.

4. McGuire WP, Rowinsky EK: Old drugs revisited, new drugs and experimental approaches in ovarian cancer therapy. *Semin Oncol* 18:255–269, 1991.

5. Muggia F, Braly PS: A phase III randomized study of cisplatin versus taxol and cisplatin in patients with suboptimal stage III and IV epithelial ovarian cancer: A Gynecologic Oncology Group study No. 132, Philadelphia, 1992.

53

Pancreatic Cancer

Overview

- ▪ Fourth leading cause of cancer deaths in U.S.

- ▪ Five-year survival trend is shifting upward toward meager 5%

- ▪ Fewer than 15% of persons are alive 1 year after diagnosis

- ▪ Difficult to detect or diagnose before it is advanced

- ▪ Accounts for 2% of all cancers and 5% of cancer deaths

- ▪ Peak incidence occurs between 45 and 60 years of age

- ▪ Japanese immigrants to U.S. have higher incidence

■ Risk factors are few

1. Occupational exposure to aluminum milling, gasoline derivatives

2. Naphthylamine, benzidine exposure

3. Tobacco

4. Diet high in fat, meat, or both

5. Peptic ulcer

■ About 95% of tumors arise from endocrine parenchyma

■ Adenocarcinoma is dominant morphologic type

■ Tumors occur twice as frequently in head of pancreas as in tail or body of pancreas

■ Pancreatic tumors grow rapidly with late signs of pathology

■ Tumor growth is often extension or spread to common bile duct

■ Metastatic spread involves regional or paraduodenal lymph nodes

Approaches to Care

■ Assessment

1. Clinical manifestations

  ❏ Early signs are vague and often referred to other organs

❏ *Head of pancreas manifests classic triad of symptoms*

   ☐ Pain

      ▪ In epigastric region
      ▪ Dull and intermittent
      ▪ Ameliorated by lying or bending forward

   ☐ Profound weight loss

   ☐ Progressive jaundice

      ▪ Appears first on mucous membranes, then palms, then generalized

      ▪ Weight loss of 20 to 30 pounds in a few weeks can occur

      ▪ Patients complain of emotional disturbances and irritability

❏ *Body of pancreas manifests symptoms late in advanced stages*

   ☐ Severe excruciating epigastric pain causes vomiting

   ☐ Hepatomegaly and splenomegaly

❏ *Tail of pancreas mimics other diseases*

   ☐ Metastases to liver, bone, lungs, peritoneum, and other organs may be first sign

   ☐ Generalized weakness

   ☐ Upper abdominal pain

   ☐ Indigestion, anorexia, weight loss

■ **Diagnostic measures**

1. Physical examination

2. **Radiologic studies: CT scan, CT-guided biopsy, endoscopic retrograde cholangiopancreatography, arteriography**

3. **Lab profiles, tumor markers (CA 19–9, CEA, POA)**

■ **Interventions**

1. **Radical therapy if cure is believed possible**

2. **Palliative therapy if disease is advanced**

3. **Surgery**

   ❏ *Plagued by low resectability rates*

   ❏ *Patients with small (<2 cm) tumors experience 30% 5-year survival rates*

   ❏ *Surgical approaches for cure*
      □ Total pancreatectomy
         ▪ En bloc resection including antrum, common duct, gallbladder, pancreas, jejunum, duodenum, and nodes
      □ Pancreatoduodenectomy (Whipple procedure)
         ▪ Resect distal stomach, pancreas to superior mesenteric vein, duodenum, proximal jejunum, distal common duct, and gallbladder
      □ Regional pancreatectomy
         ▪ Resect entire pancreas, duodenum, gastric antrum, bile duct, gallbladder, spleen, and nodes
      □ Distal pancreatectomy
         ▪ Resect only involved pancreas and nodes

❑ *Surgical approaches for palliation*
  ☐ Decompression procedures
    ■ Cholecystojejunostomy
    ■ Choledochojejunostomy
    ■ Pancreatojejunostomy

  ☐ Biliary bypass procedures
    ■ Gastroenterostomy

❑ *Postoperative care focuses on prevention of*
  ☐ Hemorrhage
  ☐ Hypovolemia
  ☐ Hypotension
  ☐ Pulmonary complications
  ☐ Exocrine and endocrine alterations
    ■ Endocrine function can be regulated with insulin

    ■ Exocrine function can result in malabsorption syndromes. Nutritional therapy, pancreatic enzyme supplements, and lipase administration may be needed

    ■ Diet therapy
      Low-fat, high-carbohydrate foods
      Small meals
      Restrict caffeine
      Restrict alcohol

4. Chemotherapy

❑ *Used as adjuvant therapy with limited results*

❑ *Agents used*
  ☐ 5-Fluorouracil   ☐ Ifosfamide
  ☐ Mitomycin-c   ☐ Doxorubicin
  ☐ Streptozotocin

5. Radiotherapy

❏ *Used for both palliative and curative external therapy*

❏ *Limitation to effectiveness is large volume of tissue to be irradiated*

❏ *Combinations of radiotherapy and chemotherapy are used successfully to increase survival time*

6. Supportive therapy: Most common measures

❏ *Continuous administration of pain relief measures*

❏ *Nutritional support via oral feedings, supplemental mixtures, antiemetic therapy, feeding tube, pancreatic enzyme replacements*

❏ *Relief of jaundice using cholestyramine, lotions, avoiding soaps*

❏ *Relief of obstruction via percutaneous transhepatic biliary drainage*

Suggested Readings

1. Frogge MH. Gastrointestinal cancer: Esophagus, stomach, liver, and pancreas. In Groenwald SL, Frogge MH, Goodman M, Yarbro CH (eds.): *Cancer Nursing: Principles and Practice* (3rd ed.). Boston: Jones and Bartlett, 1993, pp. 1004–1043.

2. Ahlgren JD, Hill MC, Roberts IM: Pancreatic

cancer: Patterns, diagnosis, and approaches to treatment. In Ahlgren JD, Macdonald JS (eds.): *Gastrointestinal Oncology.* Philadelphia: Lippincott, 1992, pp. 197–208.

3. Spross JA, Manalatos A, Thorpe M: Pancreatic cancer: Nursing challenges. *Semin Oncol Nurs* 4(4):274–284, 1988.

4. Miyata M, Nakao K, Takao T, et al: An appraisal of pancreatectomy for advanced cancer of the pancreas based on survival rate and postoperative physical performance. *J Surg Oncol* 45:33–39, 1990.

54

Prostate Cancer

Overview

■ Most common cancer in American men and second leading cause of cancer death

■ Highest rate is among black Americans

■ Cause is unknown but risk factors include

1. Age: Between 60 and 70 years of age

2. Hormonal factors: Abnormal estrogen and androgen levels

3. Family history

■ Ninety-five percent are adenocarcinomas and arise most often in posterior lobe of gland

■ Tumor growth varies from slow to moderately rapid

■ **Survival related to extent of tumor and histologic grade**

Approaches to Care

■ **Assessment**

1. Clinical manifestations

❏ *Usually asymptomatic in early stages*

❏ *Routine rectal examination reveals nodule or mass*

❏ *More than 50% of patients present with localized disease*

❏ *Common symptoms include*
- Prostatitis
- Urinary frequency
- Weak stream
- Postvoid dribbling
- Nocturia
- Dysuria
- Hematuria
- Weight loss
- Back pain

2. Diagnostic measures

❏ *Digital rectal examination*

❏ *Transrectal ultrasonography and biopsy*

❏ *Elevated prostate-specific antigen*
- Levels > 4ng/ml indicate benign prostatic hypertrophy or cancer
- Levels > 10ng/ml point to malignancy

❏ *Cytologic examination of urine and prostatic fluid*

❑ *Excretory urogram*

❑ *CT and bone scans, and MRI*

■ Interventions

1. **Treatment is controversial and varies**

2. **Four methods are used either alone or in combination**

   ❑ *Radical prostatectomy*

     □ For patients in good health with localized tumors

     □ Complications include
       ■ Impotence
       ■ Urinary incontinence

   ❑ *External beam radiotherapy*

     □ Curative treatment for localized disease

     □ Palliation for advanced disease

     □ Common side effects
       ■ Proctitis
       ■ Urinary frequency
       ■ Cystitis
       ■ Diarrhea
       ■ Incontinence and impotency

   ❑ *Endocrine manipulation*

     □ Used as palliation to reduce tumor size

     □ Most prostatic tumors are androgen-dependent; therapy attempts to block androgen formation or utilization

     □ Methods
       ■ Bilateral orchiectomy

- Hormonal agents

  Diethylstilbestrol   *Flutamide*

  Leuprolide   *Aminoglutethimide*

  Goserelin acetate   *Ketoconazole*

□ Complications
  - Gynecomastia
  - Hot flashes
  - Nausea and vomiting
  - Edema
  - Decreased libido
  - Erectile impotence

□ Eighty-five percent of patients with advanced disease respond to hormonal manipulation

□ Duration of response is 1 to 3 years

❏ *Chemotherapy*

  □ Limited role for chemotherapy in advanced, hormonally unresponsive prostate cancer

  □ Both single-agent and combination regimens are being investigated

3. Nursing interventions include

❏ *Encouraging men older than 40 years to have annual rectal examination*

❏ *Provide suggestions for managing loss of libido, impotence, loss of fertility, or urinary incontinence*

❏ *Provide postoperative care of bladder irrigations, catheter care, prevention of infection, wound management, treatment for incontinence, pain management, and sexual assessment*

❑ *Teach patient about side effects of radiotherapy, hormonal therapy, and chemotherapy*

Suggested Readings

1. Lind J, Kravitz K, Greig B: Urologic and male genital malignancies. In Groenwald SL, Frogge MH, Goodman M, Yarbro CH (eds.): *Cancer Nursing: Principles and Practice* (3rd ed.). Boston: Jones and Bartlett, 1993, pp. 1258–1316.

2. Maxwell MB: Cancer of the prostate. *Semin Oncol Nurs* 9:237–251, 1993.

▪ 55 ▪
Skin Cancers

Overview

■ **Generally occur in adults between ages 30 and 60 years**

■ **There are two groups**

1. Nonmelanoma skin cancer (NMSC)

❑ *Basal cell carcinoma (BCC)*
  ☐ Most common skin cancer in whites
  ☐ More frequent in men
  ☐ Least aggressive type

❑ *Squamous cell carcinoma (SCC)*
  ☐ More frequent in men
  ☐ More aggressive than BCC

2. Malignant melanomas

❑ *Most are cutaneous melanomas (CM)*
❑ *Primarily occur in whites*
❑ *More frequent in men*

- ■ NMSCs occur more often but have a lower mortality rate than malignant melanomas

- ■ Melanoma has high mortality rate

- ■ Etiologic factors

1. Light skin, hair, and eyes; easily sunburned
2. Ultraviolet radiation
3. Chlorofluorocarbons
4. Precursor lesions
5. Atypical and changing moles
6. Ionizing radiation
7. Hereditary conditions

Approaches to Patient Care

■ NMSC

1. Assessment

- ❏ *Nodular BCC*
    - □ Small, firm, dome-shaped papule
    - □ Pearly white, pink, or skin-colored
    - □ Ulcerates as it enlarges
    - □ Most common sites
        - Face
        - Head
        - Neck

- ❏ *Superficial BCC*
    - □ Flat
    - □ Erythematous or pink scaling papules

      ☐ Well-defined margins

      ☐ Common sites

         ■ Trunk

         ■ Extremities

❑ *SCC*

    ☐ Flesh-colored or erythematous

    ☐ Raised, firm papule

    ☐ May ulcerate and bleed

    ☐ Common sites are areas exposed to sun

       ■ Nose   ■ Back of hands

       ■ Forehead   ■ Lower lip

       ■ Ear

2. Interventions

❑ *Treatment selection depends on*

    ☐ Tumor type

    ☐ Location

    ☐ Size

    ☐ Growth pattern

    ☐ Patient age and general health

❑ *Primary goals of treatment are*

    ☐ Cure

    ☐ Preservation of tissue and function

    ☐ Minimal risk

    ☐ Good cosmetic results

❑ *There are five standard treatments for NMSCs*

    ☐ Surgical excision

       ■ Can be performed for any NMSC

       ■ Allows for rapid healing

       ■ Provides good specimen for histologic examination

       ■ Provides good cosmetic results

☐ Chemosurgery (Mohs' micrographic surgery)
  - Preserves maximum amount of tissue
  - Complex and specialized technique
  - Often used in high-risk areas (nose, ear)

☐ Curettage and electrodesiccation
  - Used for small, superficial, or recurrent BCC because of poor margin control

☐ Radiotherapy for lesions that are
  - Inoperable
  - Located in corner of nose, eyelid, lip and canthus
  - Larger than 1 cm but smaller than 8 cm

☐ Cryotherapy
  - Involves liquid nitrogen to freeze and thaw tissue; leads to tumor necrosis
  - Used for recurrent lesions, multiple superficial BCC, and lesions with well-defined margins

■ Melanoma

1. Assessment

❏ *There are three precursor lesions of CM*
  ☐ *Dysplastic nevi* (DN)
    - May occur in familial and nonfamilial settings
    - Risk of CM is 100% in members of families with familial DN
    - DN appear between ages of 5 and 8 years, with dysplastic changes after puberty

- Patient with "classic" DN has

  More than 100 moles

  One mole larger than 8 mm

  One mole with CM features

- DN appear on face, trunk, arms, buttocks, groin, scalp, and breast

- Pigmentation is irregular with mixtures of tan, brown and black, or red and pink

- Excisional biopsy is first line of treatment

- Follow-up by

  Periodic skin examinations

  Total-body photographs every 3 to 6 months

- Individuals with DN and family members should be taught

  To examine entire body every 1 to 2 months

  Preventive behaviors

  Melanoma risk factors

☐ *Congenital nevi*

- Present at birth or shortly thereafter

- Range in size from large to small, covering arms, hand, or trunk

- Colors range from brown to black

- Lesions may have irregular surface

- Lifetime risk of malignant transformation is 6% to 7%

- Treatment consists of surgical excision

☐ *Lentigo maligna*
- Large
- Tan with shades of brown
- Ten to 25 years before malignant transformation

❏ *The "ABCD" rule helps to identify CM*

A = asymmetry

B = border irregularity

C = color variation or dark black color

D = diameter more than 0.6 cm
(pencil eraser size)

❏ *Four major types of CM are*
- ☐ Lentigo maligna melanoma
  - Four percent to 10% of CM
  - Least serious type
  - Common sites are areas exposed to sun
    Face
    Neck
    Back of hands
- ☐ Superficial spreading melanoma
  - Accounts for 70% of CM
  - Seen on trunk and back in men
  - Seen on legs in women
  - Aggressive
- ☐ Nodular
  - Accounts for 15% to 30% of CM
  - Common sites are head, neck, trunk
  - Most aggressive

□ Acral lentiginous
  ■ Found in 35% to 60% of dark-skinned persons, primarily blacks, Asians, and Hispanics
  ■ Occurs on palms, soles, nailbeds, mucous membranes

2. Treatment interventions

❏ *Surgery*
  □ Biopsy for suspected CM
  □ Wide excision for stage I CM
  □ Excision of primary lesions and surgical dissection of involved nodes for clinical stage II
  □ Elective lymph node dissection is controversial

❏ *Chemotherapy*
  □ Metastatic melanoma is resistant to chemotherapeutic agents

❏ *Radiotherapy*
  □ Most effective when tumor volume is low
  □ Often used for palliation

❏ *Immunotherapy*
  □ Several agents (interferons, interleukins, tumor necrosis factors, monoclonal antibodies) are under investigation

3. Preventive interventions

❏ *Many skin cancers can be prevented by reducing exposure to risk factors*

❏ *Preventive behaviors*
  □ Minimize sun exposure, especially between 10 AM and 3 PM

  ☐ Wear protective clothing (hat, sunglasses)

  ☐ Use waterproof sunscreen with sun protective factor of 15 or more

  ☐ Protect self when near surfaces that reflect ultraviolet rays (water, sand, snow, concrete)

  ☐ Be aware of photosensitivity caused by medications

  ☐ Avoid tanning parlors

  ☐ Keep infants well protected

❏ *Early detection and diagnosis are essential*

❏ *High-risk individuals should receive periodic skin examinations*

4. Nursing interventions

❏ *Interview that questions patient's knowledge, medical history, and exposure to risk factors*

❏ *Thorough skin assessment to identify suspicious lesions*

❏ *Education about skin cancers*

❏ *Posttreatment management and follow-up*

Suggested Readings

1. Ketcham M, Loescher L: Skin cancers. In Groenwald SL, Frogge MH, Goodman M, Yarbro CH (eds.): *Cancer Nursing: Principles and Practice.* (3rd ed.). Boston: Jones and Bartlett, 1993, pp. 1238–1257.

2. Berwick M, Bolognia JL, Heer C, et al: The role of the nurse in skin cancer prevention, screening, and early detection. *Semin Oncol Nurs* 7:64–71, 1991.

3. Lawler PE, Schreiber S: Cutaneous malignant melanoma: Nursing's role in prevention and early detection. *Oncol Nurs Forum* 16:345–352, 1989.

4. Loescher LJ: Skin cancer prevention and detection update. *Semin Oncol Nurs* 9:184–187, 1993.

■ 56 ■
Stomach Tumors

Overview

■ Gastric cancer is insidious in its onset and mimics other gastric maladies

■ If detected early and treated aggressively, it can be cured

■ Overall survival rates are 16% to 92% depending on stage at time of diagnosis

■ Incidence is increasing in some parts of the world, but decreasing in U.S.

■ In U.S., there are about 24,000 new cases and 16,000 deaths from gastric cancer each year

■ Higher incidence is seen among African Americans, Japanese immigrants, Chinese immigrants, and native Hawaiians

■ **Risk factors**

1. **Environmental and genetic factors**

2. **Immigrants exhibit incidence rates similar to those of their country of origin**

3. **Those at greatest risk are older than 40 years and possess one or more of the following**
   - ❏ *Low socioeconomic status*
   - ❏ *Poor nutritional habits*
   - ❏ *Vitamin A deficiency*
   - ❏ *Family history of gastric cancer*
   - ❏ *Pernicious anemia*
   - ❏ *Achlorhydria*
   - ❏ *Chronic gastritis*
   - ❏ *Gastric polyps*
   - ❏ *Benign peptic ulcer disease*

■ **More than 90% of gastric cancers are adenocarcinoma**

1. **Most arise in gastric antrum**

2. **May be classified as polypoid, scirrhous, ulcerative, or superficial**

■ **Can progress and metastasize by several routes**

1. **Extension and infiltration along mucosal surface and stomach wall or lymphatics**

2. **Via lymphatic or vascular embolism**

3. **By direct extension into adjacent structures**

4. **Via bloodstream**

Approaches to Care

■ Assessment

1. Clinical manifestations

❏ *Vague, nonspecific symptoms, which lead to delays in seeking medical help*

❏ *Pain in epigastric, back, or retrosternal area*

❏ *Vague, uneasy sense of fullness, feeling heavy*

❏ *Feeling moderate distention after meals*

❏ *Progressive weight loss with advanced disease*

❏ *Disturbance in appetite*

❏ *Nausea, vomiting*

❏ *Weakness, fatigue, anemia*

❏ *Dysphagia*

❏ *Hematemesis, melena*

2. Diagnostic measures

❏ *Complete assessment of nutritional status and diet history*

❏ *Physical examination for abdominal mass, enlarged nodes, or hepatomegaly*

❏ *Rectal examination for metastatic deposits*

❏ *If obstruction exists, peristaltic activity moving left-to-right may be detected*

❏ *Anemia and jaundice*

❏ *Diagnostic studies include*
- ☐ Double-contrast upper gastrointestinal series
- ☐ CT scan for metastases and tumor extension
- ☐ Endoscopic gastroscopy
- ☐ Direct biopsy and cytology
- ☐ Hematologic profiles

■ Interventions

1. Localized tumors are treated for curative intent with

❏ *Aggressive surgery alone or in combination with chemotherapy or radiotherapy*

❏ *About 50% of patients are candidates*

2. Advanced tumors that are partially resectable, unresectable, or disseminated are treated with

❏ *Combination therapy using surgery and chemotherapy, with or without radiotherapy*

❏ *Palliative surgery to*
- ☐ Alleviate obstruction
- ☐ Restore intestinal continuity

3. Surgery

❏ *Resectability for cure can often only be assessed on abdominal exploration*

❏ *Operability rates are about 80%*

❏ *Resectability rates are around 60%*

❏ *Potential complications*
- ☐ Pneumonia
- ☐ Hemorrhage
- ☐ Infection
- ☐ Reflux aspiration
- ☐ Anastomotic leak

❏ *Types of surgical procedures*
  ☐ Total gastrectomy for resectable lesions located in midportion of stomach
    ▪ Entire stomach, along with supporting mesentery and lymph nodes, is removed
    ▪ Esophagus is anastomosed to jejunum
  ☐ Radical subtotal gastrectomy for lesions in middle and distal portions
    ▪ Billroth I, or gastroduodenostomy, is choice for debilitated individuals, since it is not as extensive a resection as Billroth II
    ▪ Billroth II, or gastrojejunostomy, is used if person can tolerate more radical procedure and wider resection
  ☐ Subtotal esophagogastrectomy for tumor located in proximal portion of stomach or cardia

❏ *Postoperative care*
  ☐ Potential complications include
    ▪ Pneumonia   ▪ Hemorrhage
    ▪ Infection   ▪ Reflux aspiration
    ▪ Anastomotic leak
  ☐ Gastric emptying is altered
    ▪ Potential complications are typical postgastrectomy syndromes
      Steatorrhea   *Weight loss*
      Dumping syndrome   *Diarrhea*
      Nausea   *Vitamin deficiency*
      Vomiting   *Anastomotic leak*

> - Dumping syndrome is sequela that affects many but not all patients
>
>   *Small, frequent feedings of low-carbohydrate, high-fat, high-protein foods recommended*
>
>   *Restrict fluid for 30 to 40 minutes before and after meal*
>
>   *Antispasmodics and antiperistaltics can reduce diarrhea*
>
>   *Vitamin B_{12} deficiency must be treated with replacement doses*

4. Radiation therapy

- ❏ *Gastric adenocarcinomas are generally radiosensitive*

- ❏ *Location and proximity to vital organs in abdomen restrict use*

- ❏ *May be administered in combination with chemotherapy or surgery for recurrent or advanced disease*

- ❏ *Used to augment locoregional control of residual or advanced disease*

- ❏ *Multimodal approaches can improve survival*

- ❏ *Intraoperative radiotherapy is used in Japan, but not as much in U.S.*

5. Chemotherapy

- ❏ *No specific chemotherapy regimen alone effective*

- ❏ *Combination drug therapy superior to single agents*

❏ *Combinations used most often are*
  ❏ FAM (5-fluorouracil [5-FU], doxorubicin, mitomycin-c)
  ❏ FAP (5-FU, doxorubicin, platinol)
  ❏ EAP (etoposide, doxorubicin, platinol)
  ❏ FAMTX (5-FU, doxorubicin, leucovorin)

❏ *Intrahepatic and intraperitoneal administration being investigated*

6. Supportive therapy

❏ *Nutrition therapy is problematic, either due to obstruction or dysfunction; nutritional support is nursing priority*

❏ *Lack of gastric secretory function leads to enzyme and nutrient deficiencies*

❏ *Management of pain, pulmonary complications, and dehydration*

Suggested Readings

1. Frogge MH. Gastrointestinal cancer: Esophagus, stomach, liver, and pancreas. In Groenwald SL, Frogge MH, Goodman M, Yarbro CH (eds.): *Cancer Nursing: Principles and Practice* (3rd ed.). Boston: Jones and Bartlett, 1993, pp. 1004–1043.

2. Vezeridis MP, Wanebo HJ: Gastric cancer: Surgical approach. In Ahlgren JD, Macdonald JS (eds.): *Gastrointestinal Oncology*. Philadelphia: Lippincott, 1992, pp. 159–170.

3. Cady B: Gastric cancer. In Steele G, Cady B (eds.), *General Surgical Oncology.* Philadelphia: WB Saunders, 1991, pp. 139–147.

4. Wang JF: Stomach cancer. *Semin Oncol Nurs* 4(4):257–264, 1988.

▪ 57 ▪
Testicular Cancer

Overview

■ Accounts for 1% to 2% of all cancer in men

■ Most common solid tumor in men between 29 and 35 years of age

■ Higher incidence in upper socioeconomic class

■ Improved management has increased survival rates

■ Etiologic factors

1. Cryptorchidism
2. Exogenous estrogens taken by mother

■ **Testicular tumors arise from germ tissue and are classified as**

1. **Seminoma**

2. **Nonseminomatous germ cell tumors**

■ **Metastasis occurs either by extension or via lymphatics**

■ **Young men should practice monthly testicular self-examination**

Approaches to Patient Care

■ **Assessment**

1. **Clinical manifestations**

❏ *Painless enlarged testicle*

❏ *Symptoms related to metastasis include*
   □ Lumbar pain
   □ Abdominal or supraclavicular masses
   □ Cough

2. **Diagnostic measures**

❏ *Radical inguinal orchiectomy (as biopsy)*

❏ *Radiographic studies*
   □ Chest x-ray   □ Intravenous pyelogram
   □ CT scans   □ Ultrasound

❏ *Laboratory studies*
   □ Serum alpha-fetoprotein (AFP)
   □ Lactic acid dehydrogenase
   □ Human chorionic gonadotropin (HCG)

❏ *AFP and HCG (tumor markers) aid in diagnosis, response to treatment, and detection of residual tumor*

■ Interventions

1. Treatment of *nonseminomas*

❏ *Retroperitoneal lymphadenectomy (RPLND)*

❏ *Primary chemotherapy using cisplatin-based regimen for patients with metastases larger than 3 cm*

2. Treatment of seminomas

❏ *Stage I and stage II (nonbulky) disease*

  ☐ Adjuvant radiotherapy following radical orchiectomy

❏ *Stage IIB and stage III (bulky disease)*

  ☐ Primary chemotherapy using cisplatin-based regimen

3. Nursing care includes

❏ *Fertility evaluation for man who wishes to father a child later*

❏ *Anticipation of anxiety and threat to masculinity, sexual potency, and fertility*

❏ *Assurance that loss of ejaculatory ability after RPLND is usually not permanent*

❏ *Assurance of normal sexual functioning after unilateral orchiectomy*

❏ *Monitoring and management of side effects related to radiotherapy and chemotherapy*

❏ *Education, encouragement, and emotional support help men cope with testicular cancer and its treatment*

Suggested Readings

1. Lind J, Kravitz K, Greig B: Urologic and male genital malignancies. In Groenwald SL, Frogge MH, Goodman M, Yarbro CH (eds.): *Cancer Nursing: Principles and Practice* (3rd ed.). Boston: Jones and Bartlett, 1993, pp. 1258–1315.

2. Brock D, Fox S, Gosling G, et al: Testicular cancer. *Semin Oncol Nurs* 9:224–236, 1993.

▪ 58 ▪
Vaginal Cancer

Overview

■ One of rarest gynecologic tumors

■ Accounts for 1% to 2% of gynecologic tumors

■ Peak incidence is in women between 50 and 70 years of age

■ Rates are highest in

1. Black populations
2. Low socioeconomic levels

■ Vaginal tumors are usually secondary sites of metastatic disease

■ Squamous carcinoma is most common cell type

■ Vaginal intraepithelial neoplasia (VAIN)

1. Divided into three categories: I, II, III

2. Usually seen in women treated for cervical intraepithelial neoplasia or after radiotherapy for cervical cancer

■ Vaginal cancers occur most commonly on

1. Posterior wall of upper third of vagina

2. Anterior wall of lower third of vagina

■ Tumor may spread along vaginal wall into cervix or vulva

■ Metastasis to lungs and supraclavicular nodes occurs often

■ Overall survival rate is 40% to 50%

■ There is little consensus on treatment

■ Risk factors include

1. History of human papillomavirus

2. Vaginal trauma

3. Previous abdominal hysterectomy

4. Lack of regular Pap smears

5. Age (risk increases with age)

6. Young women exposed to diethylstilbestrol

Approaches to Care

■ Assessment

1. Clinical manifestations

❑ *Abnormal Pap smear*
❑ *Abnormal vaginal bleeding*
❑ *Foul-smelling discharge*
❑ *Dysuria*
❑ *Urinary symptoms*

2. Diagnostic measures

❑ *Visual examination*

❑ *Palpation of vagina*

❑ *Pap smear (for squamous cell, not adenocarcinoma)*

❑ *Colposcopy*

❑ *Vaginal and cervical biopsies*

❑ *Chest x-ray*

❑ *Biochemical profile*

❑ *Intravenous pyelogram, barium enema*

❑ *Cystoscopy*

❑ *Proctosigmoidoscopy*

■ Interventions

1. Treatment of VAIN

❑ *Depends on whether lesion is single focus or multifocal*

❑ *Depends on size of lesion*

❑ *Local excision for single-focus lesions*

❑ *Total vaginectomy for women who failed conservative therapy*

❑ *Local application of 5-fluorouracil cream*

❑ *Laser therapy for single-focus or multifocal lesions*

2. Treatment of invasive disease

❑ *Treatment of choice is radiotherapy, especially for women with stage I and stage II disease*

❑ *Small lesions may be treated with radiation*

❑ *Larger lesions may require local and regional treatment*

  ☐ High-dose local radiotherapy concomitant with chemotherapy that has cytotoxic and radiosensitizing properties

  ☐ Surgery for early-stage disease

   ▪ *Lower vagina:* Partial or total vaginectomy

   ▪ *Upper vagina:* Radical hysterectomy and upper vaginectomy plus lymphadenectomy

   ▪ *Middle or lower vagina:* Anterior or posterior exenteration

   ▪ Since 80 percent of women develop recurrence within first 2 years of surgery, treatment may need to be palliative

  ☐ Nursing measures

   ▪ Education and support during aggressive therapies

   ▪ Excellent clinical assessments and astute interventions facilitate therapeutic outcomes

   ▪ See measures listed in Chapter 59

Suggested Readings

1. Walczak J, Klemm PR: Gynecologic cancers. In Groenwald SL, Frogge MH, Goodman M, Yarbro CH (eds.): *Cancer Nursing: Principles and Practice* (3rd ed.). Boston: Jones and Bartlett, 1993, pp. 1065–1113.

2. Chamorro T: Cancer of the vulva and vagina. *Semin Oncol Nurs* 6:198–205, 1990.

3. Aho M, Vesterinen E, Meyer B, et al: Natural history of vaginal intraepithelial neoplasia. *Cancer* 68(1):195–197, 1991.

4. Manneta A, Pinto JL, Larson JE, et al: Primary invasive carcinoma of the vagina. *Obstet Gynecol* 72(1):77–81, 1988.

Vulvar Cancer

Overview

- Disease of elderly that occurs rarely; accounts for 3% to 4% of all gynecologic cancers

- Peak incidence occurs between 70 and 80 years of age

- Usually remains localized

- Has overall 5-year survival rate of between 70% and 75% for all stages; survival is even higher for women with negative nodes

- Treatment is predominantly surgical

- Two classes

1. Invasive vulvar cancer

2. Preinvasive vulvar lesions: *Vulvar intraepithelial neoplasia (VIN)*

■ **Various premalignant vulvar conditions can progress to carcinoma**

■ **Risk factors**

1. **Risk factors of invasive vulvar cancer include**
   ❑ *Advanced age (> 60 yr)*
   ❑ *Chronic vulvar disease (VIN, vulvar dystrophy)*
   ❑ *Previous malignancy of lower genital tract*
   ❑ *Human papillomavirus*
   ❑ *Herpes simplex virus type 2 (HSV2)*
   ❑ *Chronic irritation*
   ❑ *Exposure to coal tar derivatives*
   ❑ *Medical conditions: Hypertension, cardiovascular disease, obesity, diabetes*
   ❑ *History of breast, cervical, or endometrial cancer*

2. **Etiology of VIN is unclear but suggested risk factors include**
   ❑ *Venereal disease*
   ❑ *HSV2*
   ❑ *Condylomata acuminatum*
   ❑ *Immunosuppression*
   ❑ *History of genital or extragenital malignancies*

■ **Labia are sites of 70% of vulvar cancer**

1. **Labia majora involved three times more than labia minora**

2. **Can develop in clitoris, Bartholin's glands, and perineum**

■ **Vulvar cancer**

1. **Remains localized**
2. **Is squamous cell cancer (90% of cases)**

■ **Common routes of metastatic spread**

1. **Direct extension**
2. **Lymphatic spread to regional nodes (40% of cases)**
3. **Hematogenous spread to distant sites (lung, liver, bone) is rare**

Approaches to Care

■ **Assessment**

1. **Clinical manifestations**
   ❏ *Invasive vulvar cancer*
      □ Twenty percent of patients are asymptomatic
      □ Lesions detected during routine examinations
      □ Presence of mass
      □ Growth in vulvar area
      □ Vulvar pain and bleeding

   ❏ *VIN*
      □ Fifty percent of patients are asymptomatic
      □ Vulvar pruritus
      □ Burning (*vulvodynia*)

   ❏ *Woman may delay seeking treatment, sometimes for 2 to 16 months*

2. Diagnostic measures

❏ *Invasive vulvar cancer*
  ☐ Local excisional biopsy

  ☐ Colposcopy

  ☐ Pap smear

  ☐ Complete examination of vulva, cervix, and vagina

❏ *VIN*
  ☐ Inspection   ☐ Toluidine stain
  ☐ Colposcopy   ☐ Biopsy

❏ *Metastatic work-up*
  ☐ Chest x-ray
  ☐ Proctosigmoidoscopy
  ☐ Cystoscopy
  ☐ Barium enema
  ☐ Intravenous pyelogram
  ☐ Biochemical profile

❏ *Staging is according to International Federation of Gynecology and Obstetrics (FIGO) system*

■ Interventions

1. Local disease

❏ *VIN treatment is controversial*
  ☐ Wide local excision with primary closure skin flaps or skin grafts

- Multicentric disease treatment
  - Skinning vulvectomy: Vulvar skin is excised and split-thickness skin graft is applied; requires prolonged bed rest for healing to occur
  - Simple vulvectomy can be used for elderly or those with chronic diseases

- *Laser, cryosurgery, or cautery may cause painful ulcerations that take 3 months to heal*

- *Topical 5% 5-fluorouracil, dinitrochlorobenzene, and bleomycin in daily applications cause painful, slow-healing ulcers*

2. Invasive vulvar cancer is treated with surgery

- *En bloc dissection of tumor, regional inguinal and femoral nodes, vulva, and sometimes pelvic nodes*

- *Nodal dissection can also be achieved through separate incisions in groin, rather than by en bloc approach*

- *Early lesions (<2-cm lesion with <5 mm of stromal invasion) are treated with simple vulvectomy without groin dissection*

- *Stage II and stage III lesions require extensive surgery*
  - Radical vulvectomy
  - Bilateral inguinal-femoral lymphadenectomy
  - If needed, resection of surrounding organs: urethra, vagina, anus, rectum

❏ *Stage IV disease*
  ☐ Pelvic exenteration
  ☐ Radical vulvectomy (if rectum or bladder is involved)
  ☐ Radiotherapy may be used

❏ *Possible complications after radical surgery*
  ☐ Wound breakdown, infection
  ☐ Leg edema
  ☐ Lymphocyst
  ☐ Genital prolapse
  ☐ Stress incontinence
  ☐ Thrombophlebitis

❏ *Radiotherapy can be used preoperatively to reduce tumor bulk (4500–5500 cGy)*
  ☐ Useful for poor surgical candidates
  ☐ Potential wound healing problems

❏ *Recurrence occurs in 80% of cases within first 2 years of treatment*
  ☐ Surgery is used to treat recurrence
  ☐ Recurrence of groin lesions may be treated with radiotherapy

3. Nursing measures concentrate on patient education

❏ *Explain disease and treatment*

❏ *Instruct patient in self-care*
  ☐ Address concerns about sexual functioning
  ☐ Discuss changes in libido, orgasm, coital frequency, fertility

❏ *Stress importance of follow-up*
  ☐ Discuss possibility of treatment failure
  ☐ Assess patient for anxiety, depression, changes
    in self-image or body image

Suggested Readings

1. Walczak JR, Klemm PR: Gynecologic cancers. In
   Groenwald SL, Frogge MH, Goodman M, Yarbro
   CH (eds.): *Cancer Nursing: Principles and Practice*
   (3rd ed.). Boston: Jones and Bartlett, 1993, pp.
   1065–1113.

2. di Paola GR, Belardi MG: Squamous vulvar
   intraepithelial neoplasia. In Knapstein PG, diRe F,
   Disaia P, et al (eds.): *Malignancies of the vulva.* New
   York: Thieme Medical Publishers, 1991, pp. 57–72.

3. Hacker MF: Vulvar cancer. In Berek JS, Hacker MF
   (eds.): *Practical Gynecologic Oncology.* Baltimore:
   Williams & Wilkins, 1989, pp. 391–424.

4. Ball B: Easing the shock of radical vulvectomy.
   Nursing 5:27–31, 1975.

PART VI

Delivery Systems for Cancer Care

◼ 60 ◼
Rehabilitation

Overview

◼ Helps individual learn how to adapt to effects of cancer and its treatment

◼ Principles

1. Uses interdisciplinary team approach
2. Emphasis on maximizing strengths
3. Focus on practical day-to-day issues
4. Facilitation of coping with loss
5. Family care
6. Focus on prevention in areas of high risk for complications

Approaches

■ Goals

1. **Achieving optimal functioning within limits imposed by cancer is ultimate goal**

2. **Goals can be categorized to reflect trajectory of cancer patient's experience**

   ❏ Preventive: *To prevent or reduce impact of disability*

   ❏ Restorative: *To return patient to optimal functional status*

   ❏ Supportive: *To maximize function and prevent secondary disabilities*

   ❏ Palliative: *To assist dying person and family in maximizing their independence, while providing comfort*

■ Individual needs

1. **Needs encompass many areas**

   ❏ *Physiologic*   ❏ *Social*
   ❏ *Emotional*   ❏ *Spiritual*
   ❏ *Functional*

2. **Assessment of rehabilitation needs requires**

   ❏ *Careful use of professional skills*

   ❏ *Assessment tools to assure objectivity and comprehensiveness*

   ❏ *Ongoing reevaluation and update of assessments*

■ Resources for rehabilitation

1. Organized in many ways, depending on agency's resources, flexibility, and interests

2. Elements can include

- ❏ *Comprehensive approach to addressing needs*
- ❏ *Interdisciplinary team knowledgeable of cancer and family care*
- ❏ *Coordinated services*
- ❏ *Cancer rehabilitation services or teams*
- ❏ *Case manager or specialist to coordinate team of providers*

■ Cancer rehabilitation services or teams

1. Cohesive groups of professionals working collaboratively toward common patient-centered goals

2. Team members

- ❏ *Nurse*
- ❏ *Social worker*
- ❏ *Counselor*
- ❏ *Physical therapist*
- ❏ *Occupational therapist*
- ❏ *Dietitian*
- ❏ *Recreational therapist*
- ❏ *Speech-language pathologist*
- ❏ *Enterostomal therapist*
- ❏ *Chaplain*
- ❏ *Pharmacist*
- ❏ *Psychiatrist*
- ❏ *Volunteers*

3. Coordination of care is key to effective rehabilitation

■ Delivery factors

1. Outpatient needs can be met by

❏ *Providing easy access*
❏ *Appropriate scheduling*
❏ *Coordination with ongoing cancer treatment schedules*

2. Education and support groups can facilitate rehabilitation

3. Exercise groups can maximize strength and foster social interaction

4. Survivors of cancer have special rehabilitation needs

❏ *Workplace concerns*
❏ *Sexuality and intimacy*
❏ *Body image and self-esteem*
❏ *Values and beliefs*

5. Survivor and transition groups can be helpful

Suggested Readings

1. Ferrell BR, O'Neil-Page E: Continuity of care. In Groenwald SL, Frogge MH, Goodman M, Yarbro CH (eds.): *Cancer Nursing: Principles and Practice* (3rd ed.). Boston: Jones and Bartlett, 1993, pp. 1346–1359.

2. Frymark SL, Mayer DK: Rehabilitation of the person with cancer. In Groenwald SL, Frogge MH, Goodman M, Yarbro CH (eds.): *Cancer Nursing: Principles and Practice* (3rd ed.). Boston: Jones and Bartlett, 1993, pp. 1360–1370.

■ 61 ■
Ambulatory Care

Overview

■ Has increasingly important role in cancer care

■ Eighty percent to 90% of cancer care is delivered in ambulatory setting

■ Settings include

1. Comprehensive cancer centers

2. Freestanding cancer centers

3. Twenty-four-hour clinics

4. Chemotherapy and blood therapy infusion centers

5. Day hospital clinics

6. Physicians' offices

7. Outreach and network programs

8. Specialty centers for screening, rehabilitation, symptom management

■ Nurses have complex roles

1. Direct nursing care
2. Education and counselling
3. Health maintenance and preventive care
4. Coordination of services
5. Continuity of care

Ambulatory Care Issues

■ Models of nursing care delivery

1. Primary nursing
2. Multidisciplinary teams
3. Collaborative nurse-physician practice
4. Case management

■ Patient classification and nurse productivity systems

1. Many systems have been proposed and examined, but few can capture many direct and indirect activities of nurse in these settings

■ Quality assurance and improvement

1. Ensures that care is provided at or above established standards of care
2. Patient satisfaction with care has become an area of intense interest

3. Ambulatory patients' needs and satisfactions may differ significantly from those factors nurse might identify as important

■ Occupational hazards and safety

1. Not as highly regulated as in acute setting

2. Safely handle antineoplastic agents, radioactive materials, and blood and body fluids

3. Be informed of proper practices

4. Adhere to current safety practices to avoid occupational hazards

■ Continuity of care

1. Enhanced in outpatient setting by electronic communications

2. Development of tools and documentation materials appropriate to any patient care setting

3. Critical elements for continuity
   - ❏ *Uniform access to care*
   - ❏ *Comprehensive planning*
   - ❏ *Responsiveness to patient and family needs*
   - ❏ *Availability of resources and services*
   - ❏ *Coordination of care*
   - ❏ *Monitoring quality of care*

Nurse's Role in Ambulatory Care

■ **Major elements**

1. **Admission and assessment**

2. **Patient and caregiver education**

3. **Telephone triage and counselling**

4. **Documentation of care and education**

5. **Documentation of response to treatment and education**

   ❏ *Self-care teaching and support*
   ❏ *Treatment delivery*
   ❏ *Safety*
   ❏ *Infection control*
   ❏ *Sexuality*
   ❏ *Self-esteem*
   ❏ *Ethical issues: informed consent*
   ❏ *Economic issues*
   ❏ *Insurance*

6. **Alternative sources of funds or supplies**

■ **Nurses in ambulatory care are involved in fastest growing segment of cancer care. Challenges of growth, reimbursement, volumes, acuity, care standards, delivery systems, and coordination are but a few of the issues and opportunities ahead**

Suggested Readings

1. Ferrell BR, O'Neil-Page E: Continuity of care. In Groenwald SL, Frogge MH, Goodman M, Yarbro CH (eds.): *Cancer Nursing: Principles and Practice* (3rd ed.). Boston: Jones and Bartlett, 1993, pp. 1346–1359.

2. Otte DM: Ambulatory care. In Groenwald SL, Frogge MH, Goodman M, Yarbro CH (eds.): *Cancer Nursing: Principles and Practice* (3rd ed.). Boston: Jones and Bartlett, 1993, pp. 1371–1402.

▪ 62 ▪
Home Care

Overview

■ One of most rapidly growing and changing fields in health care

■ Can be preventive, diagnostic, therapeutic, rehabilitative, or for long-term maintenance care

■ Services typically include

1. Nursing
2. Homemaker-home health aide
3. Physical therapy
4. Occupational therapy
5. Speech-language pathology
6. Social work
7. Nutrition services

■ Types of agencies

1. **Official public health agencies**

2. **Medicare-certified agencies**

3. **Private-duty agencies**

4. **Specialized services agencies: infusion therapy, durable medical equipment**

Unique Characteristics

■ Patient and family determine when and how care will be implemented

■ Patient and family assume responsibility for care

■ Environmental barriers to safe care can exist

■ Lack of utilities or facilities for providing care

■ Potential presence of vermin or hazards

■ Inadequate coverage and financial limitations are common

Home Care Issues

■ Situations that evoke stress for caregivers

1. **Managing physical care and treatment**

2. **Managing own home and patient's home and finances**

3. **Need to be available 24 hours a day, 7 days a week**

4. **Fear of leaving patient alone**

5. **Change in relationship or communications between patient and caregiver**

6. **Disruption in household routines**

7. **Preparing different meals**

8. **Inability to spend time with own spouse and children**

9. **Often trying to balance need to work outside home with care of patient**

10. **Inability to meet expectations of health care system due to lack of time, knowledge, skill, or just being overwhelmed**

■ **Most helpful nursing interventions as identified by patients include**

1. **Giving excellent, knowledgeable, skilled, and personalized nursing care to patient**

2. **Providing patient with necessary emergency measures if need arises**

3. **Assuring patient that nursing services will be available 24 hours a day, 7 days a week**

4. **Allowing patient to do as much for himself or herself as possible**

5. **Teaching family members how to keep patient physically comfortable**

6. **Answering questions honestly, openly, and willingly**

7. **Supporting cohesion of family by initiating and promoting interaction, communication, cooperation, and social and emotional involvement**

8. **Directing nursing intervention toward daily problem solving**

■ **Economic issues**

1. **Are significant struggle for home care providers**

2. **Nurses must be familiar with reimbursement guidelines**
   ❑ *Eligibility criteria*
   ❑ *Definitions of levels of service*
   ❑ *Nuances of documenting for reimbursement*

■ **Ethical concerns**

1. **Certain possessions, routines, and family structures may not be conducive to provision of care in home**

2. **Nurses develop creative alternatives or intervene carefully in adjusting environment as much as possible**

3. **Withholding treatment for personal or financial reasons are among most common issues faced**

Home Nursing Roles and Activities

■ **Direct nursing care and treatments**

1. **Completes physical examination of patient during each home visit**

2. **Demonstrates all nursing care procedures being taught to caregivers in home**

3. **Performs all procedures requring skill of nurse (administration of intravenous fluid, insertion of feeding tube, etc.)**

4. **Administers chemotherapy prescribed by physician**

5. **Obtains laboratory specimens requested by physician to monitor effects of disease or disease treatment (specimens of blood, urine, sputum, or wound cultures)**

■ **Observation and reporting of disease, treatment response, and family response**

1. **Assesses and reports signs and symptoms of emergency medical problem resulting from side effects of medical treatment of disease (e.g., bone marrow depression following chemotherapy)**

2. **Assesses and reports potential signs and symptoms of emergency medical problem resulting from tumor (e.g., hypercalcemia)**

3. Assesses and reports signs and symptoms of disease progression

4. Evaluates patient's response to prescribed medications and therapies

5. Assesses patient's and family's emotional response to course of disease and/or course of treatment

■ Supervision of self-care or caregivers

1. Identifies current and potential problems influencing patient's care, including ability of patient to obtain needed care in home

2. Plans nursing care to correct, improve, or manage identified patient problems

3. Provides written instructions of medication schedules or patient care procedures for caregivers in patient's home

4. Supervises care given to patient in home by family, friends, volunteers, or home health aides

5. Coordinates admission to hospital if need arises

■ Health and disease management teaching

1. Instructs regarding actual and potential effects of disease process based on patient's or caregiver's readiness and ability to learn

2. Teaches actual and potential effects of disease treatment on patient

3. Teaches signs and symptoms requiring immediate notification of nurse or physician

4. Teaches purpose, side effects, amount, frequency and method of administering each medication and treatment prescribed (e.g., analgesics, colostomy care, decubitus ulcer care)

5. Instructs regarding nutrition and hydration requirements, including methods appropriate for individual patient

6. Instructs regarding rehabilitation and self-care techniques (e.g., ambulation with walker, range-of-motion exercises for lymphedema, energy saving, comfort measures)

7. Instructs regarding prevention of complications and infections, including environmental safety and hygiene

8. Instructs regarding health promotion and maintenance, with emphasis on prevention and early detection of disease

■ Counselling and support

1. Identifies emotional, spiritual, or social problems experienced by patient and family

2. Assists patient and family to identify and express their feelings about effects of disease or treatments

3. Facilitates referral to appropriate resources for extended counselling

■ **Coordination and collaboration of home care community supports and medical care**

1. **Assists patient and family to utilize formal and informal support services within community**

2. **Assesses and prioritizes patient and family needs; integrates and coordinates appropriate home health services into the plan of care (e.g., home health aide, medical social work, occupational therapy, physical therapy, speech therapy, nutrition consultation)**

   (Source: Michigan Cancer Foundation Services, Inc. Home Care Program, 110 E. Warren, Detroit MI 48201)

■ **Specialized cancer care**

1. **Infusion therapy**
   - ❏ *Most rapidly growing segment within home health care*
   - ❏ *Venous access devices and pumps enable home infusions*
   - ❏ *Home parenteral infusion and home antibiotic therapy are also becoming common*

2. **Chemotherapy administration**
   - ❏ *Most common in cancer care*
   - ❏ *Often cost-effective*
   - ❏ *Other factors*
     - ☐ Criteria for patient selection must be met
     - ☐ Patient has to be able to receive chemotherapy in home

- ☐ Insurance reimbursement varies and should be thoroughly checked to avoid unnecessary financial stresses
- ☐ Procedures for administration are well documented
- ☐ Staff are educated in processes and particularly
  - Safety considerations of drug transport
  - Preparation of drugs
  - Spills
  - Patient care
  - Disposal of drugs and supplies
  - Patient and family responsibility and education

3. Pain management

- ❏ *Develop analgesic regimen that is simple to administer and provides sufficient pain relief to allow optimal functioning*
- ❏ *Ensure that pain medications given around clock, not as needed*
- ❏ *Employ measures other than analgesics consistently and effectively (e.g., relaxation techniques)*
- ❏ *Initiate interventions to prevent potential side effects of narcotic analgesic regimen concurrently (e.g., anticonstipation medications)*
- ❏ *Provide ongoing comprehensive assessment of patient's pain (identify source of pain whenever possible and do not assume that patient's pain is due to malignant process)*

❑ *Identify and dispel patient and family misconceptions about use and abuse of narcotic analgesics*

Quality Assessment in Home Care Setting

■ **Measure care with established standards for home care**

■ **Move underway to shift emphasis from measuring structure or process to examining links between processes of care and desired patient outcomes**

Suggested Readings

1. Ferrell BR, O'Neil-Page E: Continuity of care. In Groenwald SL, Frogge MH, Goodman M, Yarbro CH (eds.): *Cancer Nursing: Principles and Practice* (3rd ed.). Boston: Jones and Bartlett, 1993, pp. 1346–1359.

2. McNally JC: Home care. In Groenwald SL, Frogge MH, Goodman M, Yarbro CH (eds.): *Cancer: Principles and Practice* (3rd ed.). Boston: Jones and Bartlett, 1993, pp. 1403–1431.

▪ 63 ▪
Hospice Care

Overview

- ▪ Objective is to facilitate comfortable and natural death

- ▪ Palliative medical management is pivotal

- ▪ Relief of suffering in dying goes beyond identifying and treating physical symptoms to also addressing emotional, spiritual, and existential components of suffering and pain

- ▪ Principles of palliative care

1. Overall goal of treatment is to optimize quality of life; i.e., hopes and desires of patient are fulfilled

2. Death is regarded as natural process, to be neither hastened nor prolonged

3. Diagnostic tests and other invasive procedures are minimized, unless likely to result in alleviation of symptoms

4. Use of "heroic" treatment measures is discouraged

5. When using narcotic analgesics, right dose is dose that provides pain relief without unacceptable side effects

6. Patient is expert on whether pain and symptoms have been adequately relieved

7. Patients eat if they are hungry, and drink if thirsty; fluids and feedings are not forced

8. Care is individualized and based on goals of patient and family, as unit of care

Models of Hospice Care

■ Independent, community-based programs

■ Hospital-owned programs

■ Part of home-health agency

■ Coalition programs or nursing home programs

■ Reimbursement and funding methods

1. Two of every three are Medicare-certified to receive funding

2. Eighty percent of current hospices are operated as not-for-profit organizations

Patient Services

■ Each hospice program has its own criteria for selecting patients to receive hospice care

■ In most programs, patient must

1. Have primary caregiver

2. Reside in geographic area of providing hospice

3. Agree to palliative, not curative, treatment

Nursing and Hospice Care Services

■ Core services usually include

1. Medical director   4. Pastoral care

2. Nurse coordinators   5. Trained volunteers

3. Social services

■ Other services could include

1. Dietary counselling

2. Occupational therapy

3. Physical therapy

4. Speech therapy

5. Art therapy

6. Home health aide/homemaker

7. Psychologist

8. Volunteer and bereavement coordinator

■ Hospice nurse's role includes

1. Being experienced practitioner with specialized skill in terminal care

2. Working cooperatively and communicating effectively within multidisciplinary framework

3. Demonstrating self-direction and initiative

4. Coordinating care and services provided

5. Being leader within multidisciplinary hospice team

6. Individualizing plan of care to maximize patient's comfort

7. Ability to foster relaxed, warm, personal relationship with patient, family, and other team members

Death in Home

■ Unique to hospice is approach to death in home

■ Advantages of home death are predominantly sense of family's role in contributing to social being of family

■ Much unwanted medical intervention that would typically accompany hospitalization is avoided

■ Some caregivers may find physical and emotional tasks of providing care at home too difficult

■ Preparation of patient and family for death is emphasized by hospice team

■ Hospice team is available at all times, which is of utmost importance to family

■ Facilitating grief and providing for bereavement care are critical elements

1. Bereavement involves

   ❏ *Accepting reality of loss*

   ❏ *Experiencing pain of grief*

   ❏ *Adjusting to environment in which deceased is missing*

   ❏ *Withdrawing emotional energy and replacing it into another relationship*

2. Abnormal grief can be

   ❏ *Prolonged*

   ❏ *Masked in behavioral or physical symptoms*

   ❏ *Manifest in exaggerated or excessive expressions of normal grief reactions*

Legal and Ethical Issues Surrounding Hospice Care

■ **Advance directives require informed decision and ongoing support**

■ **Hospice supports clear and informed decision**

■ **Euthanasia and suicide contain moral, ethical, and legal questions that have remained unanswered for centuries**

■ **Hospice does not support involvement in either, but promotes treatment for cause of despair and support during process of dying**

■ **Underserved populations (poor, minorities) are also underserved by hospice programs**

■ **Active hospice staff and volunteers are attempting to broaden coverage of hospice care to underserved populations**

Suggested Readings

1. Ferrell BR, O'Neil-Page E: Continuity of care. In Groenwald SL, Frogge MH, Goodman M, Yarbro CH (eds.): *Cancer Nursing: Principles and Practice* (3rd ed.). Boston: Jones and Bartlett, 1993, pp. 1346–1359.

2. Martinez J, Wagner S: Hospice care. In Groenwald
   SL, Frogge MH, Goodman M, Yarbro CH (eds.):
   Cancer Nursing: Principles and Practice (3rd ed.).
   Boston: Jones and Bartlett, 1993, pp. 1432–1450.

PART VII

Professional Issues for the Cancer Nurse

▪ 64 ▪
Ethical Issues in Cancer Nursing Practice

General Ethical Issues in Cancer Nursing Practice

■ **Autonomy**

1. Respect for individual's freedom to make choices about treatment and care
2. Individuals are responsible for their own moral acts and must make their own moral rules

■ **Beneficience**

1. Health care professionals must act in best interest of patient

■ **Nonmaleficence**

1. To help, or at least to do no harm to patient

■ **Justice**

1. **Requires that each person is given his or her due**

■ **Compassion**

1. **Comprehension of suffering experienced by another**

■ **Termination of treatment**

1. **Withholding and withdrawing treatment**

   ❏ *Is intent hastening death, or diminishing suffering?*

   ❏ *Issues under debate are whether to legalize active euthanasia, to provide aid in dying, and physician-assisted suicide*

   ❏ *Planning for good death leads to restraint of technologic interventions at various stages in course of disease, depending on patient's values and willingness to trade possible severe side effects for chance for improved, albeit temporary, quality of life*

   ❏ *Nurses can assist families to make decisions in advance so that some control can be exerted over dying*

   ❏ *Patients have common law and constitutional right to refuse treatment even if they are not dying*

   ❏ *Ethical considerations arise when individuals are not able to make decisions on their own, and have not given prior instructions*

❏ *Many states require that advance directives be written*

□ Preferred instrument is Durable Power of Attorney for Health Care

- Names in advance individual who will speak for patient when patient is incompetent to make decisions about health care

- Limited in time to duration of incompetence

- Limited in scope to decisions about health care

□ Without Durable Power of Attorney, state may determine patient and family rights

□ Obtain advance directives from all patients, especially seriously ill ones

■ **Access to care**

1. **Some argue that health care options should be limited for elderly as means of allocating scarce resources**

2. **Ethics dictate that limits are set by whether treatment provides meaningful change in outcome for patients during last years, rather than by age**

3. **Statistics show that elderly choose highly technical interventions less often than younger cancer patients**

Guidelines for Nursing Care

■ **Duty to protect patient's life lies primarily in protecting his or her autonomy and value hierarchy**

1. **Pay close attention to discovering patient's value system through**

   ❏ *Values assessment interview*

   ❏ *Constant discussion with patient and family throughout course of treatment*

■ **Require patients to update advance directive on entering health care institution, nursing home, or hospice in accordance with current Patient Self-Determination Act procedures**

1. **Supply patients with instructions as to their right to issue advance directives, and sample forms with instructions for how to prepare them**

2. **Teaching guides should be developed to train health care professionals in process of implementing patient advance directives**

Suggested Readings

1. Thomasma DC: Ethical issues in cancer nursing practice. In Groenwald SL, Frogge MH, Goodman M, Yarbro CH (eds.): *Cancer Nursing: Principles and*

Practice (3rd ed.). Boston: Jones and Bartlett, 1993, pp. 1520–1535.

2. Thomasma D: Ethics and professional practice in oncology. *Semin Oncol Nurs* 5:89–94, 1989.

3. Taylor C: Ethics in health care and medical technologies. *Theor Med* 11:111–124, 1990.

4. Quill TEJ: Death and dignity—A case of individualized decision making. *N Engl J Med* 324:691–694, 1991.

Questionable Methods of Cancer Therapy

Overview

■ Each year more than half of the million Americans diagnosed with cancer will be cured with scientifically sound therapies

■ Each year thousands of cancer patients will use questionable cancer remedies to prevent, diagnose, or treat cancer

■ Questionable methods include diagnostic tests or therapeutic methods that

1. Have not shown activity in animal models or in scientific clinical trials

2. Do not protect consumer since they do not meet requirements of U.S. Food, Drug and Cosmetic Act

Popular Questionable Methods

■ Promoted as cure or prevention of cancer, methods include

1. Metabolic therapy (manipulation of diet and detoxification by enemas)

2. Macrobiotic diet

3. Megavitamins

4. Laetrile

5. Herbal therapy

6. Live-cell therapy (injection of cells from animals)

7. Oxymedicine (hydrogen peroxide, ozone gas)

8. Antineoplastins

9. Mental imagery

10. Immunoaugmentative therapy

11. Electronic gadgets

■ Tijuana, Mexico has become haven for unorthodox clinics

■ Promoters rely on testimonials and anecdotes

Who Seeks Questionable Cancer Treatments, and Why?

■ Limited studies report that patients who seek such therapies are

1. White

2. Educated

3. Asymptomatic

4. Experiencing advanced disease

■ Motivations and reasons for use include

1. Fears

2. Desire for self-control

3. Antiestablishment

4. Social pressures from family and friends

Control of Questionable Methods

■ Any new method of cancer treatment in U.S. must meet certain scientific standards before it receives government approval for interstate distribution

■ State governments also participate in regulation

■ **Organizations provide information to health professionals and public about questionable methods**

1. American Cancer Society, (800) ACS-2345

2. National Cancer Institute, (800) 4-CANCER

3. Food and Drug Administration, (301) 443–5006

4. Consumer Health Information & Research Institute, (816) 753–8850

5. National Council Against Health Fraud, (714) 824–4690

Nursing Interventions

■ **Identification of quackery**

1. Is treatment based on unproven theory?

2. Is there purported need for special nutritional support?

3. Is there claim for painless, nontoxic therapy?

4. Have claims been published in peer-reviewed scientific journal?

5. Has treatment been compared to placebo?

6. Are proponents recognized cancer experts?

7. Do proponents claim benefit for treatment as well as prevention?

8. Is preparation a secret?

9. Is there an attack on medical establishment?

10. Do promoters demand "freedom of choice"?

■ Be knowledgeable of risks of such methods and toxicity if patient is using them in combination with standard therapy

■ Assess communication channels and patient motivations for potential use

■ Maintain positive communication channels with patient and family who may be interested in or participating in such methods

■ Maintain patient participation in health care

■ Patient education is most powerful approach towards controlling questionable remedies

Suggested Readings

1. Yarbro CH: Questionable methods of cancer therapy. In Groenwald SL, Frogge MH, Goodman M, Yarbro CH (eds.). *Cancer Nursing: Principles and Practice.* Boston: Jones and Bartlett, 1993, pp. 1536–1552.

2. Lerner I, Kennedy BJ: *Questionable Methods of Cancer Treatment.* Atlanta: American Cancer Society, 1993.

Index